CW01176120

The Unexpected

The Unexpected

KAYTE ALEXANDER

To Pam,
May you always enjoy good health!
All best wishes,
Kayte

FLOKI PUBLISHING LIMITED

Floki Publishing Limited
www.kaytealexander.com

First published in the United Kingdom in 2022 by
Floki Publishing Ltd
Level 3, 207 Regent Street, London, W1B 3HH

ISBN: 978-1-7399972-1-2

Copyright: © Kayte Alexander, 2021
Design and Layout Copyright © Floki Publishing Ltd, 2021
Cover Image © Kayte Alexander, 2021

First Edition: June 2022

Kayte Alexander is hereby identified as the Author of this work in accordance with Section 77 of the Copyright, Designs and Patents Act 1988.

All rights reserved. No part of this work may be reproduced or utilised in any form or by any means, electronic or mechanical, including photocopying, recording or by any information storage and retrieval system, without the prior permission of the publisher.

For permission credits, see pages 275 and 276.

A Cataloguing in Publication record for this title is available from the British Library.

Printed and bound by Inky Little Fingers in the United Kingdom.

NEITHER THE PUBLISHER, NOR THE AUTHOR are engaged in rendering professional advice or services to the reader. This book is not intended as a substitute for medical advice from a licensed healthcare practitioner. Any decision involving the treatment of an illness should be made only after consulting a physician. Do not adjust your medication in any way without professional medical advice. The reader should consult his or her medical, health, or other competent professional before adopting any of the suggestions in this book or drawing any inferences from it.

The author and publisher specifically disclaim all responsibility for any liability, loss, or risk, personal or otherwise, which is incurred as a consequence, directly or indirectly, of the use and application of any of the contents of this book. Please note that the medical content presented herein is for your information only. It is not a substitute for professional medical advice, and it should not be used to diagnose or treat a health problem, disease or allergy. Please consult your healthcare provider if you have any questions or concerns.

References are provided for informational purposes only and do not constitute endorsement of any websites, products or other sources. I also cannot vouch for the absoluteness of my suggestions. Please seek professional medical advice before buying or utilising any product.

Readers should be aware that the websites listed in this book may change.

Preface

While lying in a hospital bed attached to countless machines and feeling very vulnerable, I decided if I ever managed to leave the hospital that I would write a book to help others who might find themselves in a similar, daunting situation.

My own experience of myocarditis, heart failure and cardiomyopathy has been a particularly long and arduous one. I believe there are two main reasons for this. Firstly, it took an inordinate amount of time before I received the correct diagnosis, and secondly, good information about myocarditis is extremely scarce and there are very few cardiologists worldwide who have a true understanding of the disease.

I am a great believer that knowledge is power, and by writing this book, I am attempting to help those patients, family members and medical practitioners who have been or are currently navigating the complexities of these conditions. Also, my aim is to provide the lay person with a better understanding of the workings of the heart and to share some of the information I have acquired on this journey whilst trying to recover and improve my own health.

I have occasionally found the format of some books about health to be somewhat dry and difficult to read. Therefore, I have attempted to design this book in a more accessible format: as a story, a recipe trove and an all-encompassing curation of research, personal anecdotes, and helpful suggestions to improve health and well-being.

I hope I have succeeded in this endeavour, and if I manage to help at least one other person in writing this book, it will have been worthwhile.

Note from the Author

The Unexpected is semi-autobiographical. Although it has been inspired by a true story, many of the names, characters, places and details have been changed to protect the privacy of individuals and to make for a better narrative.

Acknowledgements

I would like to take this opportunity to thank all those who have supported me throughout my journey and while writing this book – my mother and father; my family and friends; the team of cardiologists and medical practitioners who have treated me; the enduring support of the Myocarditis Foundation; and…

The Unexpected kindness of strangers.

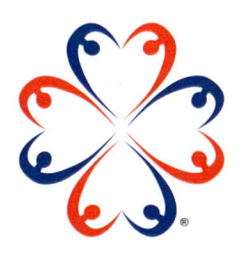

Thank You

Thank you for buying this book. Each copy sold will provide a donation to the Myocarditis Foundation.

If you have enjoyed reading it, please recommend it to others. Additional copies may be purchased directly from the website:

www.kaytealexander.com

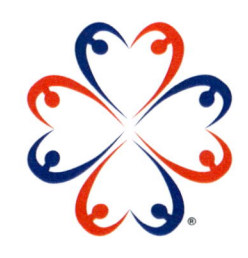

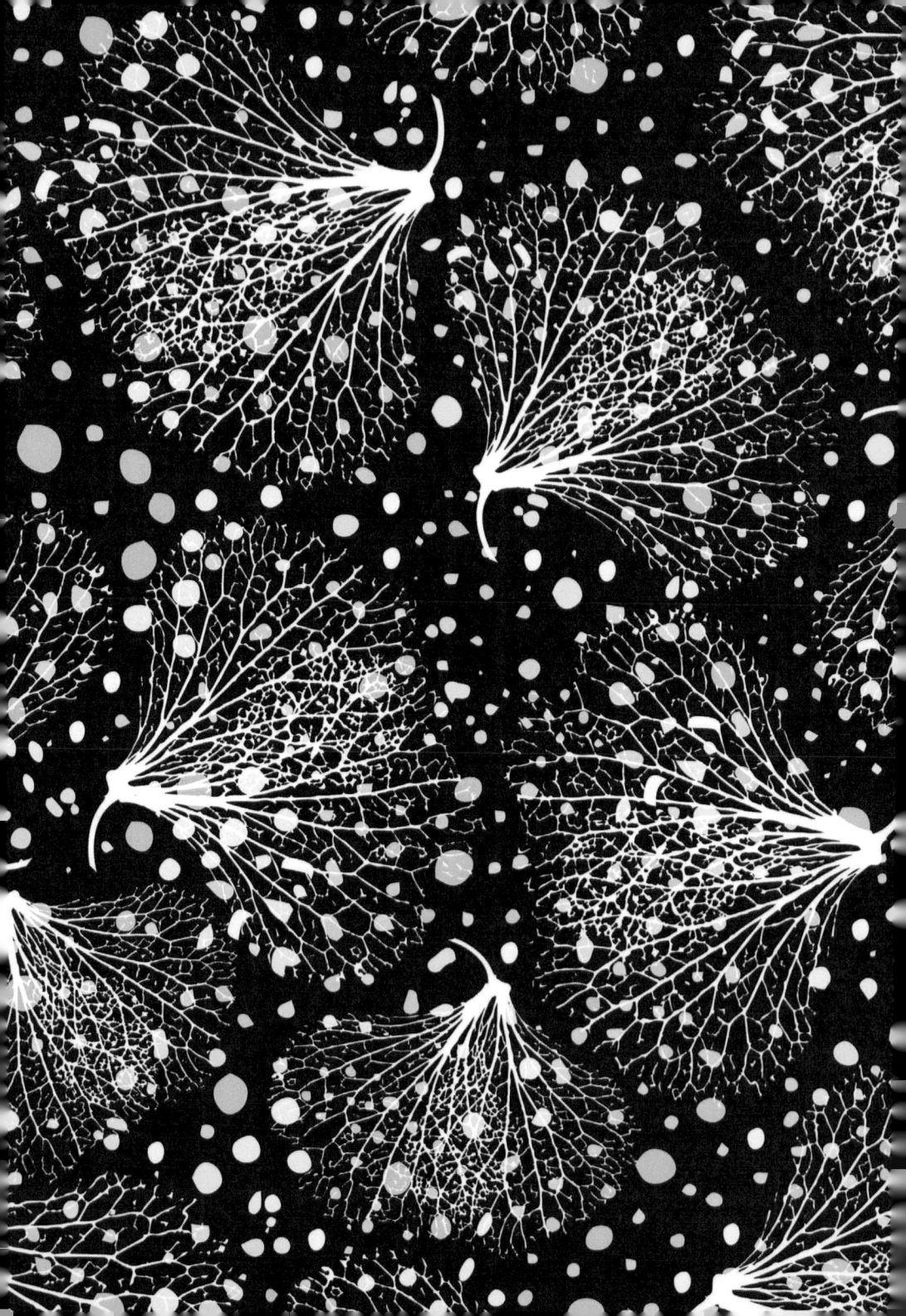

Part One

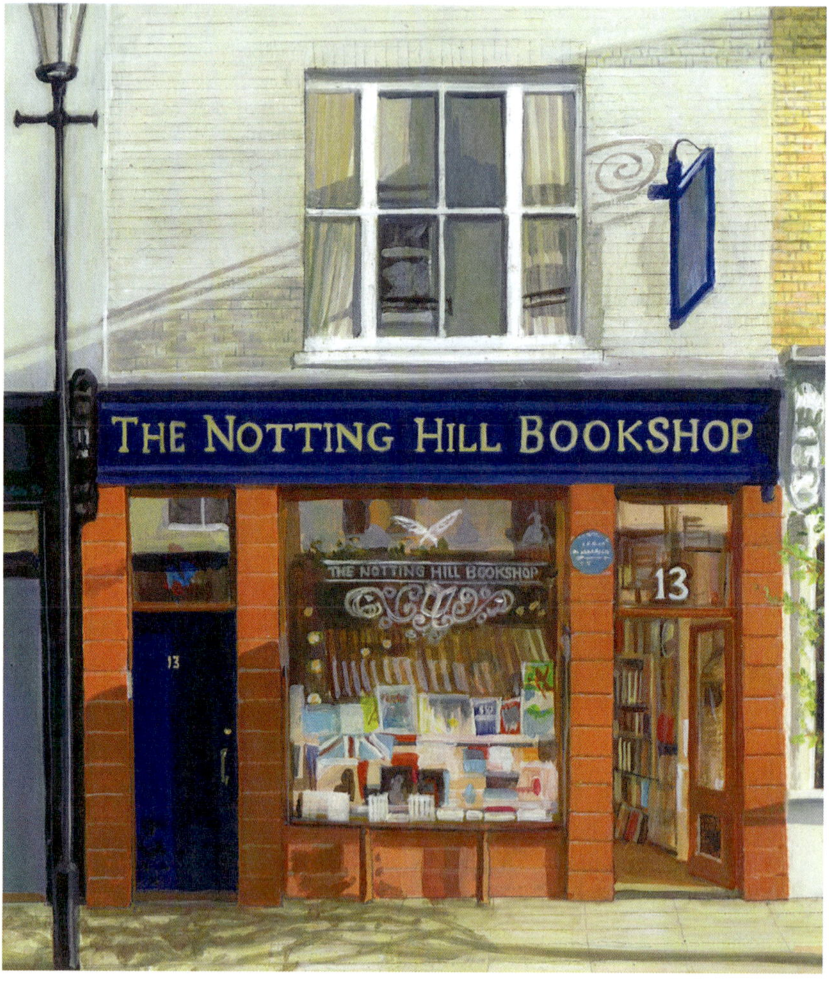
THE NOTTING HILL BOOKSHOP
THE NOTTING HILL BOOKSHOP
13
13

CHAPTER 1

"Kind words can be short and easy to speak, but their echoes are truly endless."

Mother Teresa

I moved to the bohemian neighbourhood of Notting Hill in the summer of 1997. The lush green vegetation of the numerous private gardens eased the transition from my previous home in Washington, DC, although the inclement summers and sombre winters in London proved somewhat challenging. I was fortunate to find a cheery apartment overlooking a carefully manicured private garden surrounded by exquisite, Regency-style terraced houses and have lived there ever since.

Notting Hill did not have the most salubrious of reputations when I moved there. Although it was well known for the Carnival, in certain areas it had a prolific drug scene and many of the houses were in desperate need of care and attention, often concealing their inherent architectural splendour and beauty. However, since 1999 and the delightful Richard Curtis movie, *Notting Hill*, the whole area rapidly became gentrified with bankers and hedge fund managers exchanging places with the eccentric occupants of former years. Whole swathes of local stores have been replaced by high street shops, although a few of the quirky former businesses remain, hanging on to the dream before some rich developer makes them an offer they can't refuse.

Another new addition to the area is the Saturday morning walking tour with groups of tourists trundling around the streets, following their tour guide as they seek out the famous blue door and 'The Notting Hill Bookshop' which was the inspiration for 'The Travel Book Co.' as featured in the movie, smartphones and digital cameras capturing their own personal snapshots of Notting Hill life. I often watch them from my window as they listen intently to the various gems of information emanating from their guide, ever hopeful they might bump into Hugh Grant or Julia Roberts purchasing their morning coffee.

Notting Hill still has many flavours of the past, particularly as most of the magnificent Italian Renaissance architecture was listed in 1969, preventing some monstrosity from being erected to spoil the architectural integrity. However, this hasn't stopped the mega basement from being imposed on the area and the occasional collapse of a Victorian terrace house in a cloud of dust.

In the early 1820s, Thomas Allason, an architect and landscape gardener, had a vision for the area and devised a plan which was greatly influenced by the designs of John Nash for Regent's Park. Alas, the financial crash of 1825 prevented the plans from being carried out, and curiously, in 1837, Notting Hill was briefly the site of a racecourse called 'The Hippodrome'. There are few references which remain, Hippodrome Place and the blue plaque at St. John's Church being the only two that I could find. The plot on which the church is built was formerly the grandstand, a perfect location to view the horse racing as it was situated at the highest point in the middle of the racecourse. For a variety of reasons, the racecourse was unsuccessful, lasting only three years, and the land was sold off to numerous individual property speculators for the construction of housing. Consequently, this led to a mishmash of different designs and gives the area its own unique personality. I've often mused why modern Britain continues to build identical houses in vast estates with very little green space and few trees instead of the architectural variety seen in certain parts of London and other cities around the world.

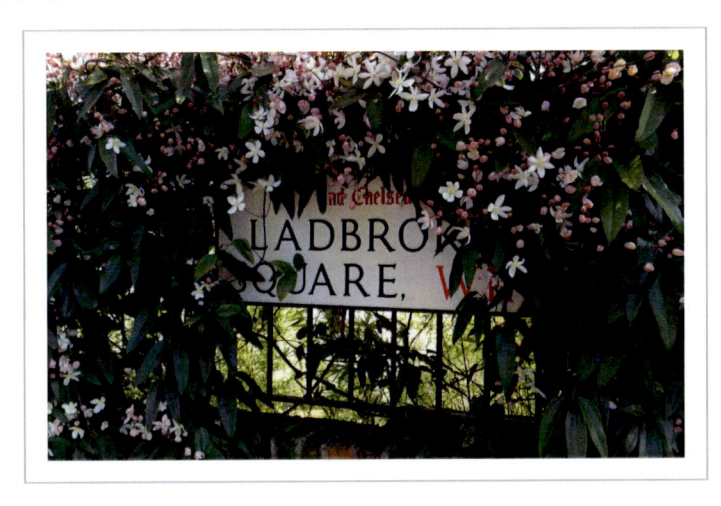

Fortunately, Thomas Allason's designs were not completely abandoned, and a flavour of his vision remains in the work of another talented architect, Thomas Allom. He designed the Ladbroke Estate comprising the most glorious Regency-style houses, beautifully landscaped gardens as well as St. Peter's, one of the last churches built for the Church of England in the Victorian classical style. Since my illness, I have grown to appreciate even more profoundly the enduring charm of the romantic architecture of the Ladbroke Estate and the architect's foresight in providing the area's residents with the most graceful private gardens, fifteen in total, and the largest, Ladbroke Square. This fragrant garden has played a significant role in my recovery as it provides a welcome haven from all the noise and distractions of London life. I have also become reacquainted with the seasons, as the changes in the garden occasionally mirror the different textures of my illness.

Life provides us with many twists and turns, and I sometimes wonder if I hadn't moved to London from America how my life would have turned out and whether all the pieces would not have lined up in such a way for me to contract a serious illness. I had been fortunate to be healthy up to this point taking great care to eat well, exercise and watch my weight. I'm not a typical candidate for a heart condition, and therein, I believe, lies one of the reasons why it took so long to reach my diagnosis and perhaps, hopefully, why I'm still here.

Life is short, we're just passing through...

A few years ago, in late spring, I had a brief business trip to New York planned and decided to make time to visit my close friend Jeff, who lived there and who had, sadly, just been diagnosed with leukaemia. Jeff had been a close friend for many years and I had a hard time coming to terms with the severity of his illness. However, he remained extremely upbeat, despite the ravages of the treatment, and was determined he would regain his good health.

I took the afternoon flight with a few colleagues on Wednesday and landed at JFK around 7pm. An enormous shiny black limousine collected us from the airport and on the way to the hotel we all decided to skip dinner and do our own thing. I checked into the charming boutique hotel we had booked on the Upper East Side. The reception staff were very friendly, and I passed the time of day with the bellman as he helped me with my bags.

'Where are you from Ma'am?' he asked.

'I've just arrived from London. It's certainly cold here, isn't it?' I replied, feeling somewhat concerned that my spring coat was a little light for the unusually cold temperatures.

'Yes Ma'am, it's one of them nor'easters. It's gonna last all weekend. Wrap up warm Ma'am, the wind chill makes it feel much colder. How's the weather in London Ma'am, still raining?' he chuckled.

'No,' I replied. 'It's been quite nice weather for the time of year. What's your name?' I asked.

'Luis, Ma'am, I'm from South Dakota,' he replied proudly.

As we reached the hotel room he opened the door, gave me a quick tour showing me all the various switches and controls, and then handed me the room keys.

'Is there anything else I can do for you Ma'am?' he asked as he hovered by the door. I was frantically trying to extract a tip from my purse and handed it to him.

'That's perfect, thank you Luis,' I said. 'You have a good evening.'

'My pleasure Ma'am. You enjoy your stay now.' He replied as he smiled and closed the door.

I was so relieved that my colleagues had felt the same way about skipping dinner. We had to attend an early morning conference the following day and I felt quite weary after the long flight, as well as a tad chilly. I switched off the air conditioning which was blasting freezing cold air into the room and decided to warm myself up by having a relaxing bath. I would then order room service and have an early night, excited at the thought of seeing my dear friend Jeff on the Thursday afternoon.

I went into the bathroom, which was surprisingly well

lit and saw a futuristic, steep-sided stand-alone bath in one corner of the room. A small jar of lavender salt with rose petals was perched on a shelf near the edge. I turned on the water which cascaded at speed from a gleaming waterfall spout and poured in some of the fragrant elixir. Changing out of my clothes, I put on the hotel slippers and a plush towelling robe that was hanging behind the door. Despite the enormous pressure of the New York water supply, the bath was so incredibly deep that it was taking quite some time to fill. Whilst waiting, I thought I had better check my emails in case there might be some 'crisis' back in the office or missive from my boss, Nigel, which needed my immediate attention.

I was still a little preoccupied by a recent occurrence at a company board meeting. I had entered the room to pass a message to one of the board members while Nigel, looking like a frog that had swallowed a bumblebee, was grandstanding about being able to treat staff badly in times of recession as they would be desperate to hang on to their jobs. I felt uncomfortable but smiled as I passed the note to Frank Willard, whom I had not seen for quite some time as he resided in New York. Nigel immediately fired a comment at me,

'What are YOU smiling at?' he said acerbically.

'Just being friendly,' I replied and then left the room. Nigel appeared to be drunk on hubris, and I could only hope that any fair-minded person would have been outraged at such boorish behaviour – a privileged, powerful man abusing his position.

As I finished scrolling my emails, I realised I was in luck. It all seemed relatively calm in London, and as the time difference was in my favour, I let out a happy sigh and grabbed my smartphone so I could find some soothing music to accompany my bath. I adjusted the temperature of the water and switched off the tap. As I lowered myself in, the fragrance from the potion enveloped my senses. I stayed there bobbing around for quite a while listening to a relaxing album by Enya and savouring the tranquil moment.

Looking back, it is at this point I realised something abnormal had occurred on that very first night at the hotel. I had relaxed in the warm water for about half an hour, topping up with hot water from time to time, but as I tried to exit the bath, I found it almost impossible to lift myself up. I sank back down and then gathered all my strength to lift myself up again. This happened three times before I finally had the thought to lower the level of the water and, luckily, I was finally able to stand up and step out. I felt quite shaken by the whole experience but put it down to some sort of strange vacuum which was applying downward pressure due to the shape and depth of the bath. I made a mental note to take a shower thereafter. However, it is very possible that my heart was already starting to struggle, and I was totally unaware.

I awoke the following day feeling refreshed, slipped on my robe and slippers, and having ordered room service for breakfast the night before to coincide with my alarm, it arrived within a few moments. I sat at a little table near the window munching on fresh berries, nuts and yoghurt while watching the US news and looked out of the window. It was a beautiful day with a clear cerulean sky and the sun was starting to reflect rainbow streaks off the glass building opposite. I checked my emails again and replied to the more urgent ones. It was incredible just how many emails had piled into my inbox overnight in such a short space of time. Nigel's emails would pour seamlessly into my mailbox mixing with my own, and it was not uncommon to receive around 300 emails every day. Consequently, the only way I could keep on top of matters was to check my BlackBerry continually. As Nigel was currently in Paris visiting his paramour, I was hoping I might get to enjoy my brief stay in New York fairly uninterrupted. I took a shower, dressed, and styled my hair which seemed to be unusually cooperative. I took particular care in getting dressed as I would be seeing Jeff later. He was such a visual person and always appreciated sartorial elegance.

The morning's meeting took place in the hotel's conference room. There were some 50 participants, and it all went off without a hitch. After lunch, I hopped into a yellow cab and made my way to Jeff's apartment, stopping on the journey briefly to buy something for afternoon tea. It was a first-floor walk-up with a small terrace in a leafy neighbourhood. I remember pressing the buzzer, and then suddenly feeling tentative, having not seen Jeff since his diagnosis. He released the catch and I walked up the ten steps to the mezzanine level. Jeff opened the door, invited me in and then we stopped and hugged briefly. I noticed that he had lost a significant amount of weight and his complexion was pale with a slight yellow tinge, his usual, sparkling deep brown eyes had faded and his hair looked a little sparse from the chemo. At that moment it dawned on me how serious his condition was, but I tried not to dwell on it and was determined to make the most of our time together. He was a fascinating man, being both a highly skilled cosmetic dentist and a mixed media artist. His apartment was decorated with many pieces of his work, and while he made us tea, I walked around examining any new creations.

'This is gorgeous!' I said, as I stood in front of a painting of a big red apple. Inserted throughout the sweeping curves were skyscrapers, symbolic of living within the Manhattan

'The Big Apple' Jeff Golub Evans

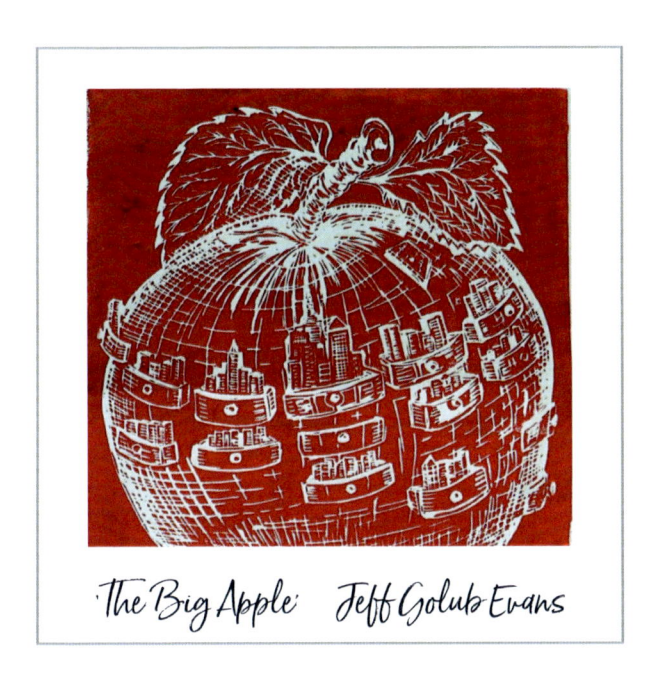

skyline. It was beautifully styled and very striking.

'Ah, that one was featured in the *New York Times* style section recently,' he confirmed. The New York-inflected tone of his voice was reassuring and reminiscent of our many conversations.

'You take just milk, right?' he called out from the kitchen.

'Yes, that's perfect, thank you. I've brought us something nice to go with our tea,' I said, as I walked back towards the kitchen carrying a beautifully designed green carrier bag containing an exquisite, highly decorated, rose-coloured box.

On a previous visit to New York Jeff had invited me to the 'Ladurée' tearoom, which had just opened on Madison Avenue. We had particularly enjoyed the 'Ispahan', a delicious rose-flavoured macaron filled with rose petal and lychee cream and embellished with fresh raspberries. As he opened the cakes and placed them on the two plates, he gazed at me for a moment then smiled and said,

'I will always love you Kayte!' His words moved me so profoundly that I suddenly felt myself tearing up. The idea that I might lose my dear friend was unbearable.

He came over and gave me a tender hug and we stayed motionless for a while cherishing the occasion whilst not uttering a sound. Looking back, I now realise that, at the time, I would not yet fully understand the significance of that special moment.

Jeff went back into the kitchen, placed all the items for tea onto a tray and carried it into the living room. There was a small dining table next to the fireplace with two chairs and we sat, munching on the cakes and drinking several cups of tea, while remaining there chatting for a few hours. Conversation with Jeff had always been so effortless. I remember meeting him for the first time, some twenty years ago, and feeling like I'd always known him. As we now lived an ocean apart, we didn't see each other frequently any more, but it was always so easy to pick up again where we had left off.

We said goodbye around 6pm and I took a cab back to the hotel. Jeff was going to get the train back to Connecticut where he lived with his family at the weekends, using the little apartment in Manhattan as a pied-à-terre while working in his dental surgery. I quickly showered and changed at the hotel and then joined my colleagues for dinner. It had been an amazing day, and although I felt somewhat tired, the infectious energy of New York invigorated me.

On the Friday, I worked in my room for most of the morning, coordinating with London and replying to emails. Earlier that morning I had received a call from one of the company's executive directors, Frank Willard, a well-mannered South Carolinian, who had a wealth of integrity and fine manners. Of all the years I had dealings with him, I never once saw him lose his temper. He was the consummate diplomat.

'Hello Ms. Kayte, how are you?' he asked, as I picked up the phone. He often called me Ms. Kayte, a Southern custom which I found rather endearing.

'Hello Frank,' I said, both surprised and pleased to hear from him. 'It's lovely being in New York,' I continued. 'How are you?'

'Well, I was wondering, Ms. Kayte, if I may take you for lunch today,' he replied. 'A little bird told me you might be free. You choose the venue. I'll take you anywhere you would like to go. It will be my treat as a thank you for all your hard work!'

Frank was set to retire from the UK executive board in a couple of months and had no plans to return to London for the foreseeable future. We settled on 'Asiate' which had a spectacular view of Manhattan and agreed to meet there at noon. I finished my emails and took a brief cab ride to Midtown.

As I arrived at the restaurant, the maître d' escorted me to a splendid table overlooking Central Park where Frank was already seated, drinking a tall glass of champagne. The restaurant had enormous floor to ceiling windows and our table was bathed in the most vivid light.

'Hello Frank, so lovely to see you,' I announced as we greeted each other.

'Hello Ms. Kayte, what a fabulous choice!'

As we passed the time of day and studied the menu, I felt quite touched that he had reached out to me and invited me to lunch. He put me at ease, taking the time to find out what I had been doing before working with Nigel, and we spent a good moment exchanging some of life's experiences.

After we had eaten the main course, his tone became a little more serious, yet empathetic.

'How are you getting on my dear?' He asked seeming genuinely interested in my reply. 'I've been a bit worried about you.' Kindness and a gentle sense of mischief mingled on his soft brown eyes.

Lately, I had often been on my guard in the office and had buried my feelings. Nonetheless, I knew that Frank had witnessed a few unfortunate scenes with Nigel at work and most recently at the board meeting. I wondered what the subtext was and considered that he might now be opening up as he was about to leave the company. Nevertheless, I was careful in my response.

'That's kind of you to notice, Frank,' I started cautiously. 'I must admit there are times when I don't understand why Nigel behaves the way he does. It seems to make life unnecessarily difficult.'

'Well, you know my dear, I don't think Nigel really likes women,' he announced unexpectedly.

I looked at him in disbelief and he smiled back understandingly. I felt relieved that someone with such integrity had noticed what was going on in the office.

'You have such a great personality; you would be a real asset to anyone who hired you,' he said generously.

'That's very kind of you, Frank,' I said softly, feeling rather lost for words.

We sat chatting for quite a while longer and then the time came for us to depart. It was such a pity he was leaving the company as he had been one of the few genuinely kind people on the board who didn't have a huge ego and was respectful of others.

I thanked him for lunch and said goodbye, not knowing if I would ever see him again. I reflected on what he had said and appreciated his concern. There have been a few other occasions in my career when someone has reached out to me unexpectedly in kindness, and again on this occasion, I felt like I had a guardian angel watching over me.

On Saturday, the sun had stopped shining. There was a heavy white sky making the weather seem even colder with very unusual temperatures for the time of year. I stepped out for a walk with a couple of colleagues in Central Park but found it very uncomfortable as, despite wearing the most luxuriant, fur-lined gloves, the circulation in my hands was cutting off with 'Raynaud's syndrome', a condition I had developed a few years earlier. As a walk was out of the question, I decided to spend the rest of my last day inside warm buildings, buying a few gifts for the London office and meeting up with my colleagues in the bar of the hotel for a drink just before we all returned to London.

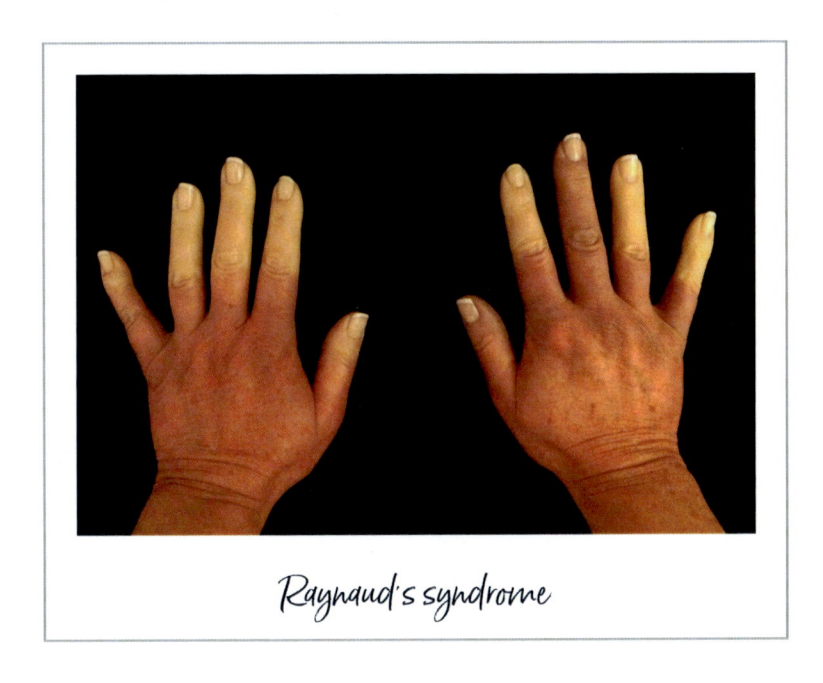

Raynaud's syndrome

CHAPTER 2

"Working to fulfil someone else's needs or dreams almost always catches up with you."

Jack Welch

The flight home was incredibly bumpy, and the severe turbulence heightened my usual anxiety of flying and prevented me from sleeping. After landing in London on Sunday morning around 7am, I ambled leisurely through the terminal at Heathrow, hopped into a black cab and when I arrived home went to bed for a couple of hours until about mid-day. The remainder of Sunday was uneventful. I spent the time catching up with friends and family, as well as checking emails before the inevitable return to the office on Monday morning.

I slept quite well that night but as I drove to work the following morning, I felt a little trepidation. As I was ahead of schedule, I took my time from the car park to the office, leisurely strolling along the pavement in the morning sunshine, which was dappled by the trees overhead. The office building was a low-rise townhouse in a London suburb, and I had been climbing the four flights of stairs to reach my office comfortably for the last seven years. However, on that morning, I reached the top of the stairs and suddenly developed a searing pain in my ribs. It was unbearable, almost as though I was being squeezed with a strap around the top of my chest. I was breathing very heavily and felt extremely odd. I remained motionless for a few moments holding on to the rail, uncertain what was happening to me. I thought of angina as I was sufficiently aware of the condition to recognise the symptoms but dismissed it as improbable at my relatively young age. I put it down to jet lag or perhaps to the onset of a chest infection. After a few moments, I regained my composure and started walking at relatively normal speed towards my office at the other end of the corridor. I passed by Pandora, the Chief Operating Officer, who was sitting in her office talking on the phone and gave her a little wave as I sauntered past. My PA, Emma, was talking to Sophie, Pandora's PA, as I entered the office suite. I smiled and announced that I had brought back some treats from New York for us to enjoy for our elevenses. As the strange symptoms at the top of the stairs had rapidly subsided, I put it to the back of my mind.

'Did you have a good time?' they asked enthusiastically.

'How was your friend?' Sophie asked thoughtfully.

'It was a great trip thank you,' I said, 'and so lovely to see my friend again,' not divulging too many details.

'It was absolutely perishing though!' I added. 'I ended up having to buy a new coat!'

I smiled knowing they would find it rather amusing as I remembered spilling something on my trousers one day at work and they thought it hilarious that I had gone out at lunch to buy another pair.

'Where's Nigel and Cindy?' I asked, noticing that their offices were unoccupied.

'Oh, Nigel's at a breakfast and then has another meeting in the City so I don't expect him until after lunch,' Emma replied nonchalantly, 'and Cindy is running a bit late,' she added, smirking.

Cindy was often late, but it never bothered me as it gave me some quiet time to prepare for the day uninterrupted and a chance to catch up with what had happened in my absence, before the inevitable arrival of Nigel, aka Baron Nigel Fetherstonhaugh III. He had one of those quirky English surnames which is pronounced completely differently from the way it is written and was pronounced quite simply 'Fanshaw'. Cindy was somewhat tempestuous, and one never knew what mood she would be in from one day to the next. I got on well with her most of the time, but occasionally she could be unpredictable and quick to lose her temper.

'It's lucky Cindy did that anger management course,' I remember jesting with Emma one day as Cindy started yelling and I was pretending to hide under the desk as a way to defuse the situation and make light of it.

I suggested to Sophie that she invite Pandora to join us for elevenses. It was unusually relaxed in the office as Nigel's heavy presence had not yet imposed itself on the atmosphere and I was still feeling invigorated from my trip to New York. Although Pandora had a good sense of humour, she also had a ruthless streak, and it was very important to keep on the right side of her. She had recently been through a rough patch herself with Nigel after he hired someone new which had diverted all his attention. Pandora had even started to wander aimlessly around the office calling herself the 'Chief Obsolete Officer', as most of her work had been reassigned, her humour masking her vulnerability, and she had lost her prized 'flavour of the month' position, an observation I kept to myself. However, when that new hire proved to be a disaster after just three months, Nigel quickly relented and brought Pandora back into the fold. Her humility was not to last, and she reverted to her usual ruthlessness and reliance on 'The Bank of Nigel'.

Nigel was CEO of a waste management company with subsidiaries in France, China, and the US. His complex character was a mass of contradictions, at times charming and at others unrelentingly combative and manipulative. He had decided that he suffered from a variety of ailments, including an aversion to the smell of food, which meant that no one in the office was allowed to eat lunch at their desks. When we did manage to go out for lunch, he would not respect the need for a break and would constantly call up and find excuses for us to return immediately. As you might anticipate, this environment did not lend itself to calm and relaxing digestion. Nigel also had an imaginary claustrophobia and used it as a reason why he couldn't sit in the middle of a row at the theatre, insisting on having the best seats wherever he went. However, this didn't correlate with his frequent airplane trips when the claustrophobia miraculously evaporated, only to return when booking theatre tickets.

Looking back, I realise just how toxic that working environment was and how many staff members were affected by it. It hadn't always appeared that way. In my job interview, Nigel had been very skilled at presenting himself as well-mannered and professional, managing to keep up the pretence for quite some time, but eventually his true character came to the fore. In reality, he was a master manipulator and a narcissist. As we all sat in glass-fronted offices, I started to observe more and more of his bullying behaviour. He would often yell at staff, his oversized hands slamming on the desk and his face, red in anger, with an errant vein swollen and visibly pulsing on his forehead. Undoubtedly, when a control freak loses control, all one is left with is the freak, but Nigel was convinced of his own moral rectitude, despite reality.

If the opportunity presented itself, I would sometimes act as gatekeeper to help vulnerable staff members avoid Nigel's ever-changing moods. Many would come to my office or meet me after work to ask my advice. Of course, I didn't realise at the time that this emotional contagion was taking its toll on my own health. I often felt like an awkward, reluctant observer while watching the next victim go through the inevitable treatment. Cindy took it all in her stride as she had worked for him since her early twenties. She was fearless and quite happy to announce that she knew where the bodies were buried if anyone dared to question her position.

Eventually my disquiet at his behaviour grew as I witnessed more and more of it, and perhaps my disdain had started to break through my protective shell, as one day he turned his sights on me and I became the next target to bully. Constructive dismissal was one of the methods he used to move people on when he grew tired of them, and I had already noticed he was starting to do this to me. I was resolute but it was often counterproductive as each time I stood my ground he became even more disagreeable. Bullies will often prey on a weakness in their quarry, and particularly as he now appeared to have noticed the Raynaud's, he would insist on having the air conditioning at full blast all year round. Consequently, sitting in Nigel's office wearing a coat was not unusual. He made a point of maintaining his office at morgue temperatures as it discouraged staff and visitors from outstaying their welcome. I would surreptitiously stop the air conditioning as I entered the room and quickly turn it back on again as I left, but I was not always successful at being undiscovered, which invariably led to some sort of backlash.

I popped out later to grab a bite for lunch and sat outside on a bench in the sunshine briefly chatting to my mother.

'I'd like to leave my job,' I announced mid-conversation. 'I just don't feel very well, and Nigel is becoming more and more obnoxious. Do you think you and Dad might help support me for a couple of months so I can have a really good rest and then look for another job?'

I had already decided to go on a trip to Washington, DC, to celebrate my upcoming birthday and had planned to hand in my notice when I returned. It had been impossible to look for another job while I was working there, as I had almost no time to breathe.

'Of course, darling,' Mum said sounding concerned. 'Dad and I have been rather worried about you lately.'

My family had a strong work ethic, and I knew my father would be concerned that I was going to be giving up a well-paid job, but my mother had observed the non-stop interruptions and relentless stress I had to contend with when visiting them on various weekends, and she was happy to give me their blessing.

I felt uplifted as I walked back to work after my conversation, in the knowledge that an end was in sight. As I entered the office suite, I noticed Nigel and Cindy were sitting in his office chatting. He seemed to be in a reasonable mood after his tryst in Paris and I popped my head around the door to say hello.

'Hello Kayte, how was the New York conference?' he asked and before I had a chance to reply, he answered a phone call and shooed us out.

As the weeks went by, I started to notice that I was getting remarkably out of breath and found it very strange. It was particularly bad when walking up the slightest slope or climbing a flight of stairs and these symptoms were getting gradually worse. I would arrive at colleagues' desks breathing heavily as though I had been out jogging. I certainly wasn't used to feeling this way, having been the fastest runner in my school and having always walked at a rapid pace. With hindsight, I now realise that subconsciously I had started making life easier for myself as I was taking cabs instead of walking from the car park or parking my car on meters closer and closer to work.

One particular day Nigel called me into his office. I had just walked upstairs from the Finance Department and was visibly panting.

'You're out of breath!' he announced in an impatient and uncaring manner.

'Yes, I know,' I replied defensively.

He was in an extremely bad mood and proceeded to launch into a tirade about the press finding out about one of his business dealings. For the first time I observed Nigel looking vulnerable, distraught, and diminished somehow. Although he was well-connected, he had been very skilled at keeping clear of the media. However, on this occasion, something must have slipped through. It seemed Nigel did have an Achilles heel after all.

As I went back to my office, it dawned on me that my symptoms were far from normal. I had always been quite resilient to stress, but this time I didn't seem to be able to cope with the slightest pressure and felt decidedly unwell. The muscle under my left eye was constantly twitching and my mouth was sore from recurring mouth ulcers. As I languished in front of my computer, I wrote a private email to my doctor, taking care not to use the company's email system. I had learnt never to use corporate email for personal matters, because too often in my working career I had seen it used as an easy excuse to fire people.

> Dear Dr. Noble,
>
> Are you around this week? I am having some funny symptoms. I first noticed it on a trip to New York a couple of weeks ago. I wasn't sure if it might be the very cold weather, but I felt quite breathless while walking outside. I have since noticed feeling breathless on a small amount of exertion e.g., climbing the stairs at work and walking up a slope. Seems a bit strange.
>
> Best wishes, Kayte

I received a reply almost immediately.

> My dear,
>
> Please make an appointment to see me as soon as possible. We must sort this out.
>
> Yours ever, Philippe

I had known Dr. Noble since my late twenties when I had worked for another company, and he was their company doctor. He was not an ordinary GP, more of an internist, as the Americans would say. He was extremely thorough, and I felt confident I would be in good hands. Making an appointment for the following day, I chose a time which might escape interruptions from the office. During the visit, he listened intently to my heart and took my blood pressure. There was absolutely no indication of any problem with my heart from the stethoscope examination and my blood pressure was reassuringly low, another red herring in all of this. Fortunately, he was sufficiently intrigued to refer me to a cardiologist.

CHAPTER 3

"It is health that is real wealth and not pieces of gold and silver."

Mahatma Gandhi

A week went by before I managed to get an appointment to see the cardiologist. I left work and picked up my car, which was parked on a meter near the office and drove across town to his consulting rooms. Dr. Ephelides was an interventional cardiologist and had an excellent bedside manner, something that I discovered subsequently is often sadly lacking in this specialty. After reading the referral letter and listening to my symptoms, he said,

'I think you might have something called syndrome X. It's a type of microvascular angina. This seems to tie in with your symptoms during cold weather and your Raynaud's condition. We'll do a full blood screen and an exercise echocardiogram to investigate a bit further. I would particularly like you to see Professor Kendall, but I believe he's currently on holiday, so you may have to wait a little while.'

He didn't seem overly concerned, but while I was sitting there listening to him Nigel interrupted by calling me on my BlackBerry. Although it was already 8pm, Nigel had always felt entitled to call me at all hours of the night and day. I switched off the phone and apologised.

'I think this is part of the problem,' I said. 'I'm under constant pressure and I'm finding it more difficult to cope than usual.' Dr. Ephelides looked at me over his reading glasses and smiled.

'Maybe it's time for you to make some adjustments,' he replied.

'Yes, I'm planning to do just that,' I said emphatically, thinking about my forthcoming holiday.

I went off to the phlebotomist for the blood tests and received the results a few days later but, unfortunately, they provided absolutely no clues. However, at this stage I was not to know that the tests carried out did not include the essential ones: cardiac troponin T and NT-proBNP. While walking back to my car, I called Nigel.

'Hello Nigel, sorry I couldn't speak just then. May I help you with something?' I said, hoping that I wasn't going to receive a verbal tsunami down the telephone.

'Yes, I need to make some changes to my speech for tomorrow. Are you in front of your computer?' he asked, sounding slightly more agreeable than usual.

'No, I've just had a blood test, but I should be home in about 20 minutes. Would that work?' I replied.

'Yes,' and he ended the call abruptly. Nigel never said goodbye at the end of a telephone conversation. I wasn't sure if it was his way of gaining the upper hand or if he just did it just for effect.

As the days went by and I waited for the exercise echo appointment, life in the office carried on as usual. I regularly worked late and decided it would be a good idea to tidy up my affairs, knowing that I would be handing in my notice after my holiday. One evening as I was just leaving the office, I encountered a security team sweeping the premises for possible listening devices, an indication of Nigel's mounting paranoia.

I managed to conceal my health concerns from my colleagues but nonetheless had mentioned to Emma that I was going to have some further tests with a cardiologist. She was a kind girl and looked concerned.

On the Thursday evening, I made my way to the hospital for the echocardiogram. I changed into a pair of trainers and sweatpants as part of the test would be on a treadmill. As I made my way to the test suite, I bounced along the corridor, the cushioning of my trainers propelling me forward and providing me with a false sense of security and agility.

Oh, I'm alright, I remember thinking to myself as I hopped along.

There's nothing wrong with me. I probably just need to do some more exercise and get fitter, I thought.

As I entered the test suite, I was surrounded by three health professionals, a professor, a registrar, and a technician. I think the professor took one look at me and must have thought I was there for a corporate health check as he left the room and went outside to speak to a colleague. The technician started the treadmill and I proceeded to walk normally while the registrar took my blood pressure. Within two minutes he had moved the treadmill to an incline, and within only a few seconds of walking uphill, I started to resemble a horse that had just completed the circuit at Ascot racecourse.

'Are THESE your symptoms?' exclaimed the technician as he gazed at me in disbelief. 'Can you manage another 40 seconds?' they said in chorus, the blood draining from both of their faces.

'Yes, I think so,' I panted, trying my best to keep up the pace.

He went running from the room as the registrar desperately tried to take another blood pressure reading. The professor reappeared, looking rather startled and perhaps feeling guilty that he hadn't been in the room when all this had occurred. He hurriedly stopped the machine and quickly moved me to the couch to lie down. I registered the shock in his voice as he took the controls of the echo machine.

'Your heart isn't pumping properly. In fact, when you're exerting yourself, it's hardly pumping at all!' he exclaimed, his voice almost squeaking.

'Is it perhaps because I'm not fit?' I ventured, hoping there might be some mundane reason for my current predicament.

'Well, I'm not fit, but my heart wouldn't be doing this,' he replied matter-of-factly.

'When are you seeing Dr. Ephelides?' he asked, looking very concerned.

'Actually, it's tomorrow evening,' I replied.

'That's good, I will speak to him before your appointment,' he concluded.

I got dressed and made my way home feeling somewhat perplexed as I had absolutely no frame of reference to draw upon. Nevertheless, I was still hopeful my cardiologist would be able to provide me with a more sensible explanation. I thought of calling my parents, but they were on holiday, and I didn't want to trouble them unnecessarily, particularly as I didn't have a definitive answer.

The following day I went back to work trying not to fret about the cardiologist appointment looming later that day. I made a concerted effort to finish any outstanding work and cleared my desk as though I was going on holiday. By good fortune, Nigel was still overseas and had been surprisingly quiet. I had a brief chat with Emma when we had a tranquil moment and confided in her.

'It didn't go very well last night, Emma.' She looked up from her work and listened intently. 'I think it's quite serious so I might have to take some time off work to get better.'

'I'm sorry to hear that,' she said, a little lost for words.

Little did I know that this would be my very last day in the office.

As I arrived at Dr. Ephelides' consulting rooms my mobile started to ring. Someone was trying to reach me from the office. I sent the call to voice mail and took a seat in the waiting area. The nurse called my name and escorted me into the doctor's office. As I entered the room, he appeared rather solemn and concerned, which is never a good sign. His youthful expression had been replaced by a rather clenched frown and he looked very serious as he announced the results.

'It's not good news, I'm afraid. Your heart is under significant duress and what you have is very serious.'

My mobile phone started ringing again, adding to the poignancy of the moment. It was another person from the office and this time I switched off the phone completely.

'But what do I have?' I bleated, almost in disbelief, the colour of the room becoming whiter and whiter and the doctor's voice trailing off further and further into the distance.

'We need to do some further investigations, more serious and invasive this time – an angiogram and an MRI – and I'm signing you off work indefinitely,' he said. His words pierced me like a needle, sudden and sharp.

Signing me off work indefinitely... I repeated the words in my head. *...angiogram.*

As I registered the word angiogram, my mind went spinning off to the case of a very dear friend, Harry, who had become seriously ill after that very procedure. The closure device (a plug sometimes used to stem the bleeding) had become infected and he had ended up in intensive care. I came back to earth with a bump and couldn't quite believe this was happening. I had absolutely no experience of this condition whatsoever to call upon. How could a perfectly healthy individual suddenly develop a problem in their heart and at such a young age?

'Could it be a virus?' I muttered, vaguely recalling an article about it some years ago in the newspaper.

'Well, it could be,' he said, 'but it's not acting like a virus!'

He confirmed that his assistant would be in touch to arrange the procedures. I shrugged on my jacket in a complete daze and left the clinic in disbelief.

As the days went by and I waited for my next appointment at home, I tried to reassure myself that I might just need something simple, like an angioplasty or a stent. One often hears of all the wonderful procedures that are now performed on the heart, and I hoped it would all turn out to be an unfortunate temporary blip. Although I had been signed off work, I still received regular emails from the HR department, no doubt instigated by Nigel, to keep up the pressure on when I might return to the office. Emma and Cindy would also call from time to time with work questions, but for the most part they left me in relative peace, and I was grateful.

Out of the blue, one evening, I received a call from Frank Willard, who had been in contact with the office and discovered I was off sick.

'Hello Ms. Kayte, I hear you're not doing too well,' he asked, sounding concerned.

'Oh, hello Frank, that's kind of you to call. Yes, the doctors don't know what's happening so I'm having an angiogram tomorrow and then an MRI in about a week's time. It's all a bit of a mystery,' I answered, feeling appreciative that he was reaching out to me.

'Don't worry Ms. Kayte, I've had one of those angiograms myself and I'm sure they'll get you fixed up in no time.'

I was grateful for his optimism, but I was beginning to realise that it might not be something that simple after all. As I was particularly worried about the angiogram procedure and the risk of infection, my friend Serena, Harry's wife, accompanied me to the clinic. Whilst walking together we both observed that my walking speed had decreased significantly as we strolled from the car to the entrance. I had to stop every few steps to get my breath back and my gait had decreased to geriatric pace.

I checked into the hospital and went with Serena to my room. Dr. Ephelides popped his head around the door and before long I was in the cath lab. The cardiologist was very skilled and explained everything as he went along. He made a small incision at the top of my leg and expertly inserted the catheter into the femoral artery. He threaded the wire along and injected contrast dye through the catheter so that he could take X-ray images of the blood vessels.

'Well, you have the coronary arteries of an 18-year-old,' he cooed, as he finished the procedure.

'That's certainly not the problem,' he added assuredly.

He applied pressure to the puncture wound in the lab and I took over the responsibility as I was wheeled back to my room. He had allowed me to use the old-fashioned procedure of applying pressure so that I might avoid any risks associated with a closure device. At least that was one less thing for me to worry about. As I returned to my room, I felt exhausted holding the cotton pad against my femoral artery and Serena took over for a short while until the bleeding had stopped. We stayed a few hours to make sure all was copacetic and then Serena took me home to rest. The next hurdle would be the cardiac MRI.

As I waited again for my next appointment, I tried to remain positive, spending the days eating lunch in a leisurely way, something I hadn't done for years, and going for a daily walk. I now know that I should have been resting at home and not putting any strain on my heart, but no one knew what was going on or had any advice to offer me.

My oldest friend, Maria, suggested accompanying me to the MRI appointment and I jumped at the chance. I wasn't sure what to expect but just having her with me was very comforting. Maria is petite with fine features, porcelain skin and sensitive blue eyes. We had been through a lot together, sharing a flat in Brussels when we started our first jobs, and latterly, she had come to stay for a short spell in London as she recovered from an acrimonious divorce.

I'm not particularly claustrophobic but wasn't looking forward to the MRI examination. As we arrived at the hospital, I left Maria in the waiting room and entered a side room where they planned to insert two cannulas before I entered the machine. I changed into a ridiculous hospital gown, with openings in the most inappropriate places. Unfortunately, the nurse couldn't manage to insert either cannula and had to call a doctor for assistance. The room had been freezing and the stress combined with the low temperature in the room had encouraged my veins to go on strike and they had disappeared into the depths. Not only did I have icy-white freezing cold hands and feet, but I was perspiring so heavily that my hospital gown became drenched. Eventually, as the doctor had only managed to insert a single cannula, he decided to use just the one.

I asked the nurse for a change of gown before moving into the MRI suite where the temperature was even lower. Luckily, I had brought along some ski socks and gloves to wear whilst inside the machine. I lay down on a very narrow, rigid table which they could slide in and out. A heavy contraption was strapped to my chest, which would allow them to see my heart in greater detail, a set of headphones fitted onto my ears and a rubber ball placed in my right hand to squeeze if I wished to speak to them. As they slid me into the MRI machine, I could feel the edges of the tunnel on both sides of my arms and if I strained my head back I could see a small opening at the very end which allowed a modest amount of light and air to penetrate the tunnel. I must admit it did feel like I was in a coffin. The rounded ceiling above me was only about six inches away, and I kept putting my head back in an attempt to get more air and to quell the anxiety that was starting to mount. I needed all my mental resolve to stay calm and motionless. I decided to close my eyes as I was not allowed to move from this point forward.

As the machine started to whirl into action, the technician's voice came through the headphones. She went through the instructions and told me I could squeeze the rubber ball at any time if I needed to speak to them. Just at that point, the ball slipped out of my hand, and I started to panic as I attempted to retrieve it.

'Breathe in, breathe out, hold…… Breathe again,' the automated voice began as I tried to get into a rhythm.

I could hear all sorts of very strange noises, and it often sounded at times like a pneumatic drill in unison with someone playing the maracas, interspersed with the Pat Metheny CD I had brought with me, supposedly to keep me calm. Breathing in at the correct moment was becoming more and more difficult as I tried to keep up with the automated voice that was firing commands over the speaker system inside the tube.

'Breathe in, breathe out, hold…… Breathe in…… breathe out, hold…… don't move, don't breathe, breathe away.'

At times I had to press the rubber ball to intervene so that I could catch my breath as I felt like I was hyperventilating and needed time to regain my composure. It was interminable and quite unpleasant. After about an hour, someone came into the room to inject me with the first substance, 'adenosine', which allowed the operator to examine the blood flow to the heart under stress. I could feel my heart protesting as I started having ectopic heartbeats all over the place. They continued scanning me for what felt like hours and then finally at the very end injected me with 'gadolinium', a contrast agent which allowed them to see the pictures more clearly. As they squeezed the substance into my cannula and left the room, I could feel the cold gel going around my system as the machine started up again with its familiar cacophony of sounds. Finally, after more than two hours they slid me out of the tube and removed all the paraphernalia. I felt incredibly stiff and breathed a sigh of relief.

As I left the suite and entered the changing room, I could hear an elderly gentleman, who had entered the MRI tunnel just after me. With great fear in his voice, he was shouting that he had to get out of the machine, that he couldn't hear what they were saying and couldn't breathe. It appeared that they had pulled him out of the machine, but he refused to go back in. I couldn't help thinking that there must be a better way.

As I was getting changed, a bubbly woman popped into the changing room with a clipboard.

'Hello, would you be willing to take part in a gene study by donating some blood before they remove your cannula?' she asked, quite oblivious to what I had just endured.

Perhaps another day I would have been more willing to help, but I felt completely spent and just wanted to get home. The cannula was removed, I got dressed and found

Maria who had been waiting patiently for me and was on her third cup of tea. She took one look at me and whisked me into a black cab. I had the most terrible headache and felt quite poorly. Maria made me a delicious supper and put me to bed, before going home. It's at times like these that good friends mean so much.

The next day I woke up feeling drained and looked very pale. The MRI had been quite an ordeal and I had to visit the cardiologist later that day to get the result. My parents had returned from vacation and were going to come and stay with me so they could be with me for the next appointment. I remember feeling a cold, clammy sensation across my abdomen as I got dressed for the appointment. The slightest exertion while putting on my clothes rendered me totally exhausted and out of breath. We arrived at the hospital, and I waited with my parents in the waiting room until my name was called. Mum and Dad stayed outside while I entered the room and sat in front of Dr. Ephelides. I felt my spirit grow heavy with anticipation.

'It seems you have severe fibrosis in the left ventricle, and it looks like you have a condition called scleroderma,' he announced.

I felt totally stunned and had never heard of this illness before. Whilst he went through the charts, I realised just how daunting it was. As he escorted me to the door, I muttered,

'Is there any risk I might pass away in the night?' wondering if it were safe for me to go home.

'I don't think you're at risk of that,' he said. 'Try to get some rest and I will come back to you when I have more information.'

I then had the unenviable task of relaying all this complicated information back to my elderly parents. I couldn't quite believe it. Whatever is scleroderma and how do you get it in the heart?

We returned home and my mother cooked dinner while I started to research the disease on the internet. As I scoured the web for information, I realised that I had none of the other symptoms of the disease, somewhat reassuringly, apart from Raynaud's and therefore I couldn't understand how they had come to that conclusion, or perhaps it was a flawed syllogism. I wrote Dr. Ephelides an email asking if scleroderma was a definitive diagnosis or possibly something else because it just didn't seem to fit with my symptoms. He replied the following day and clarified,

'You have a left ventricle with disease that looks like a ventricle with scleroderma or some variant thereof. I have consulted a disease muscle specialist for his opinion, but he thinks an endomyocardial biopsy would be a waste of time as they only provide non-specific histology findings. Let's get the rheumatology opinion first and take things from there.'

Unfortunately, this plausible hypothesis explained the symptoms and was falsely reassuring. I now know that the longer one delays the more heart muscle is damaged.

Heart Action as a Fraction

Your heart's pumping ability is often assessed using an ejection fraction. Ejection fraction (EF) is the percentage of blood your heart pumps out (or ejects) with each beat. A normal ejection fraction is between 55% and 75%. People with systolic heart failure usually have a lower ejection fraction.

My Results

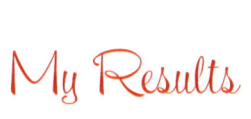

Ejection Fraction: 42%
Cardiac High Sensitivity Troponin T: not tested
BNP (NT-proBNP): not tested

CHAPTER 4

"In the sweetness of friendship let there be laughter and sharing of pleasures. For in the dew of little things the heart finds its morning and is refreshed."

Kahlil Gibran

Sometimes when you feel at your wits' end, a little something special happens to set you on a different path. Whilst I was out on my morning walk in Notting Hill, my mobile phone rang, and I heard a very welcome voice.

'Hola Dino. Qué pasa?' Joaquin announced with his deep, mellow Argentinian accent.

It was my friend, Joaquin Pascual, a professional polo player, whom I had known for many years. Not long after we first met, he had fashioned a little pet name for me, thought it was hilarious, and sported a mischievous grin every time he uttered it. He decided that I should be called 'Dino' after the Spanish word for dinosaur ('dinosaurio') because, according to him, I was so old! At first, I was rather offended to be called Dino, especially by such a good-looking younger man. He had the most beautiful smooth skin, was tall and fit with the warmest velvety brown eyes. Nonetheless, I decided to find it rather endearing as he enjoyed my company (and cooking) despite my age and of course always took great delight in beating me at Scrabble. Up to that point, I had never really thought of Joaquin as one of my closest friends, but he was funny and playful and seemed to understand me. It had always been amusing to spend time with him and to hear about his many adventures, the added benefit of his youth and vigour helping me feel young and vibrant once again. However, I always considered we were just casual friends, and I could never have expected what was about to transpire.

'Well actually I'm not very well,' I began. 'The doctor has signed me off work indefinitely.' I could feel the wind blowing wildly as I stood on a street corner in the brilliant sunshine listening to his words.

'Are you at home, Dino?' he added.

'No, but I'll be there in about 20 minutes,' I replied.

'I'm coming to see you!' he stated in a determined fashion.

No sooner had I returned to the apartment than the doorbell was sounding. Removing his shoes at the door, Joaquin entered barefoot into the living room and plopped himself down opposite me on the soft blue sofa. He had a warm glow to his skin from the Argentinian sunshine.

'What's happening Dino?' he asked, looking concerned, his velvety brown eyes watching me intently.

'Well, they're not entirely sure. It's something to do with my heart, it's not pumping properly, and they don't know why,' I explained.

'Oh dear,' he said and gazed at me for a few moments before announcing unexpectedly,

'Well, I can't help you with many things, but I do have good friends who are doctors and cardiologists in Argentina, and I will help you until you get better!'

Joaquin's kind words were like a soothing salve, and I felt totally uplifted. Suddenly the burden of my predicament seemed lighter and more hopeful. We set about putting together some of my medical reports; Joaquin translated them into Spanish and sent emails to his cousin, 'Dr. House' and to a cardiologist friend, 'Dr. Love'. Of course, these are pet names too, but I've come to realise that one should be honoured to receive a pet name from Joaquin, as it's a term of affection.

While we sat chatting on the sofa, he told me about his decision to get married. He had been dating an Italian girl for about two years, but nonetheless it was quite a step for him as he hadn't shown any interest in settling down before. He appeared to be adjusting to this newfound responsibility and was looking forward to starting another stage of his exciting life.

'Goodbye, Dino,' Joaquin said, as he gave me an enormous hug and left the apartment.

He was genuinely moved by my predicament, and despite all the arrangements for his upcoming marriage, he made a point of checking on me, and I really appreciated the sentiment. Joaquin would call me every day to see how I was doing, and I was able to observe a truly caring and gentle side to his personality. I suppose at the back of my mind I was uncertain that he would be there for me. I'm always surprised when I can count on someone, but as the days and weeks passed, all that changed, and he became the rock that I needed.

Throughout my life I have been extremely fortunate to have met some wonderful medical professionals and some have become my closest friends. I've always found medicine fascinating; perhaps it was a missed vocation, or perhaps it was because I lived with a French family whilst studying at university in Provence where both husband and wife were doctors. I was also extremely fortunate to have an unusual doctor in Brussels, who had trained as a herbalist as well as a traditional GP and was always looking for more acceptable alternatives for healing disease. Coincidentally, when living in Washington, DC many years ago, I lived opposite George Washington Hospital and consequently many friends were medical students who lived in my building and are now fully qualified doctors. Whatever the reason, I had developed a curiosity about medicine and was keen to gather information to help others. Now I needed help myself. I felt very fortunate to receive so many calls in those early days with offers of assistance from Los Angeles, New York, Washington, DC, and Texas, from Brussels and Paris and most importantly from Argentina. It was wonderful and so reassuring.

I have often been fascinated by the different ways people meet by chance and form friendships. Some years ago, when I was in my twenties, I met a rather unique character in Stuttgart while I was working there. He was a protocol officer in the US Navy and spoke several languages fluently. His name was Capt. Jay Coupe and by chance I was seated next to him at a staff dinner. He was quite an extrovert and loved to recount his numerous adventures. In the middle of dinner, he stood up and sang 'Nessun Dorma' much to everyone's delight and amusement. We had an interesting conversation, but I never thought it would lead to any further connection.

A few years later, I changed jobs and moved back to Washington, DC. My former boss, Louis, had also left Brussels and was working on Capitol Hill. One evening after work, I took out the letters from my mailbox and noticed something unusual. A white envelope stood out amongst the regular letters and bills. It was a heavy bond envelope and had been deftly addressed by a confident hand using a fountain pen. I opened the seal flap and noticed a rich gold lining. Inside was a single white card elegantly edged in gold and beautifully printed.

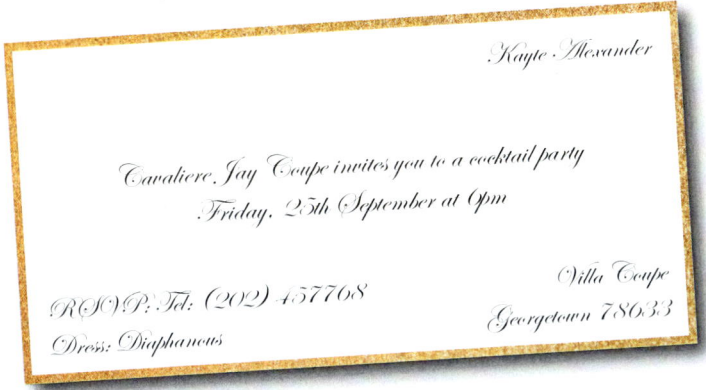

> *Kayte Alexander*
>
> Cavaliere Jay Coupe invites you to a cocktail party
> Friday, 25th September at 9pm
>
> RSVP: Tel: (202) 457768
> Dress: Diaphanous
>
> Villa Coupe
> Georgetown 78633

I read the card several times but had no idea who had sent it. I called the number on the RSVP and a slightly familiar voice answered.

'Hello.'

'Hello, this is Kayte Alexander calling. Thank you for your kind invitation for cocktails,' I said, 'but who are you?'

'Ah my dear,' he chortled. 'We met at dinner in Stuttgart a couple of years ago, do you remember?'

He went on to say that he had bumped into Louis Lightfoot in the street and asked what had happened to me. Louis had informed him that I was now living in Washington, DC. I thought I had better reply in the affirmative lest I insult him further, thanked him for the invitation and agreed to attend.

As I arrived at the Georgetown townhouse the following week, a butler answered the door, gave me a glass of champagne and I climbed the steep stairs to the first floor. The walls either side of the staircase were adorned with numerous photographs of Jay shaking hands with various dignitaries.

Oh, I remember that guy! I thought to myself, faces always being easier to recall than names. Jay was the perfect host and he introduced me to some very interesting and unusual guests. It was a friendship that would last until his untimely death some years ago. A lasting memory was Jay's ability to bring together all sorts of fascinating people, and that brief encounter would prove to be significant in my pursuance of a remedy.

On one of Jay's visits to London, I had met Alecia and her husband Ben at Harry and Serena's house. Alecia had been an eminent anaesthesiologist in Los Angeles, having trained in Hong Kong and London before moving to the US. She had a vast knowledge of all aspects of medicine and was very keen to help me. She called every few days and made thoughtful suggestions as to what I might do and whom I might see. It was apparent that the doctors I had consulted were completely baffled by the illness and the symptoms I was experiencing.

Unfortunately, as the days passed, I felt more and more weak and unable to walk about comfortably. I was referred to a rheumatologist and he checked me out for numerous connective tissue diseases, but all the results came back negative. It got to the point where it was becoming more and more difficult even to hold the phone and speak to my friends comfortably, almost as though the blood was having problems going upwards. It was also impossible to sleep on my left side. I decided to go to an IT store to buy a headset so I could talk on the phone with less discomfort. I parked the car 100 yards from the building, but it was on a slight incline. As I walked towards the store, I felt my heart shimmering and swaying in my chest.

It's getting worse, I thought to myself as I tried to avoid the passing shoppers who jostled me, unaware of my failing health. One person even rushed past me and said,

'Dead people walk faster than you do.' A comment which only added to my distress.

I bought the item and returned home as quickly as I could muster. As soon as I walked through the door of my apartment Alecia was calling and I was able to plug in the newly purchased headset.

'Hello Kayte. How are you feeling?' she asked.

'Actually, I think I'm getting worse Alecia,' I said, now starting to get increasingly worried.

We talked about whom I might go to see for a second opinion, looking up several hospitals on the internet together. However, as luck would have it, shortly after the call, I received a message from my cardiologist and he had decided to refer me to Dr. Schwarz, a pulmonary cardiologist who specialised in connective tissue disorders of the heart. He had made me an appointment for the following day.

As my plans to go on vacation to Washington, DC, and meet up with old friends had all been cancelled, I had a quiet dinner with a former colleague, Rupert, at a local Italian restaurant. It was an enjoyable evening and he introduced me to a delicious Italian wine called Falanghina. When I arrived home and popped to the bathroom, I noticed two enormous carotid arteries palpitating rapidly, high up in my neck.

'I don't think that looks normal, do you?' I said showing Rupert the pulsing sausages above my collar.

'When are you seeing the doctor?' he said.

'Tomorrow,' I answered.

'Well, that's a relief,' he replied.

The next morning, I arrived at the hospital at 8am and parked in the car park. I winced at the price, £20 an hour.

Oh well, hopefully it won't take too long, and I will soon be home again, I thought to myself.

I walked into Dr. Schwarz's office and handed him the many studies, reports, and letters that I had brought with me, hoping they might be of some use. He had a thick mop of black hair, a pale complexion and seemed a very serious individual, his manner somewhat cold and stern. After reviewing the paperwork, he looked up and said,

'Have you had a pulmonary test, a walking test, a troponin T and NT-proBNP test?'

'No,' I replied, 'I haven't had any of those tests,' as I started to wonder why they had not been performed up to now.

'Well, I'd like you to complete those tests and we'll be doing another echocardiogram here also.' He acted confident, and now I was hopeful I might finally be getting somewhere.

I spent most of the morning carrying out the various tests and at around noon the phlebotomist performed my blood work.

'You're not allowed to leave the hospital until we get the results,' the secretary informed me brusquely by telephone.

'But I'm so hungry,' I bleated, wondering how much longer this was all going to take.

'Well, you can get a bite to eat but don't go far and keep your phone with you,' she said as a compromise.

I was not to know at the time, but a failing heart needs adequate fuel and without it, like a car, will start to backfire, produce ectopic beats and feel uncertain and uncomfortable in the chest. Of course, all this was new to me, and I put it down to just hunger.

I wandered off to the high street and found a friendly Italian restaurant. Ordering a plate of pasta and a bottle of San Pellegrino, I felt much better for eating lunch. When I left the restaurant, I went for a gentle stroll around the neighbouring shops. The sun shone enthusiastically, and it was pleasing to be away from the hospital environment. As 4pm was approaching, I decided to go to a quaint English tearoom for dessert and ordered afternoon tea and a few scones. At the very moment I was about to pop one of the luscious scones with clotted cream and strawberry jam into my mouth, my mobile phone started to ring. It was the cardiologist's secretary.

'We've got the results of your blood tests back and we're admitting you immediately. You need to go to the hospital straight away,' she said excitedly. I spluttered and sent the powdered icing sugar from one of the scones over the table in a fine mist.

'What?' I said in disbelief, 'but why?' I muttered, my voice starting to falter.

'You could have a cardiac arrest at any moment,' she said matter-of-factly.

I couldn't quite believe what I was hearing.

'But I can't go straight away,' I continued, remembering my car was still in the garage, each minute that went by adding £s to my bill.

'But I need to get some belongings from home and make arrangements, I just can't leave everything,' I pleaded.

'What time can you be back?' she asked insistently.

'Well, I guess around 6pm' I suggested, hoping to make sense of all this and secretly hoping I would be able to talk to someone who would prevent a hospital admission.

She reluctantly agreed and rang off. I sat there briefly in disbelief. I had been walking around looking at cashmere sweaters only minutes beforehand and now I was being admitted to hospital, and who knew for how long. I decided to ring Dr. Noble to see what he thought.

'They're admitting me to hospital immediately,' I told him, starting to sob.

'My dear, you must do what they say,' he replied. 'Try not to fret, you will be in safe hands.'

I finished the call and rang my parents immediately to tell them. They were shocked and concerned, but it appeared to be the only option. I paid the bill quickly and made my way in a trance to the car park.

On the way home, I called Joaquin and he answered immediately.

'Are you OK Dino?' he asked tentatively. The tears welled up and I could barely speak.

'They're admitting me to hospital,' I uttered, sobbing heavily, words now escaping me.

'Are you scared?' he said. I had not considered that emotion before. However, it was evident that this was now very serious, and I wasn't improving but rapidly going downhill.

'Don't worry,' he reassured me, 'I'll come and visit you tomorrow.'

As I entered my road, I looked for a parking space where I might leave the car for a few days. As luck would have it, my neighbour was walking past, and she kindly took my keys in case the car needed to be moved. I had arranged to meet a friend, Luciana, at my flat to help me put together my overnight bag. It had now become apparent that even small tasks were beyond my capability. I made a few more phone calls to prepare for this unplanned absence and my friend Rupert kindly offered to meet me at the hospital so we could check in together.

My Results

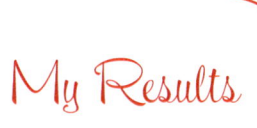

Ejection Fraction: 35%
Cardiac High Sensitivity Troponin T: 121 ng/L
BNP (NT-proBNP): 9200 ng/L

50

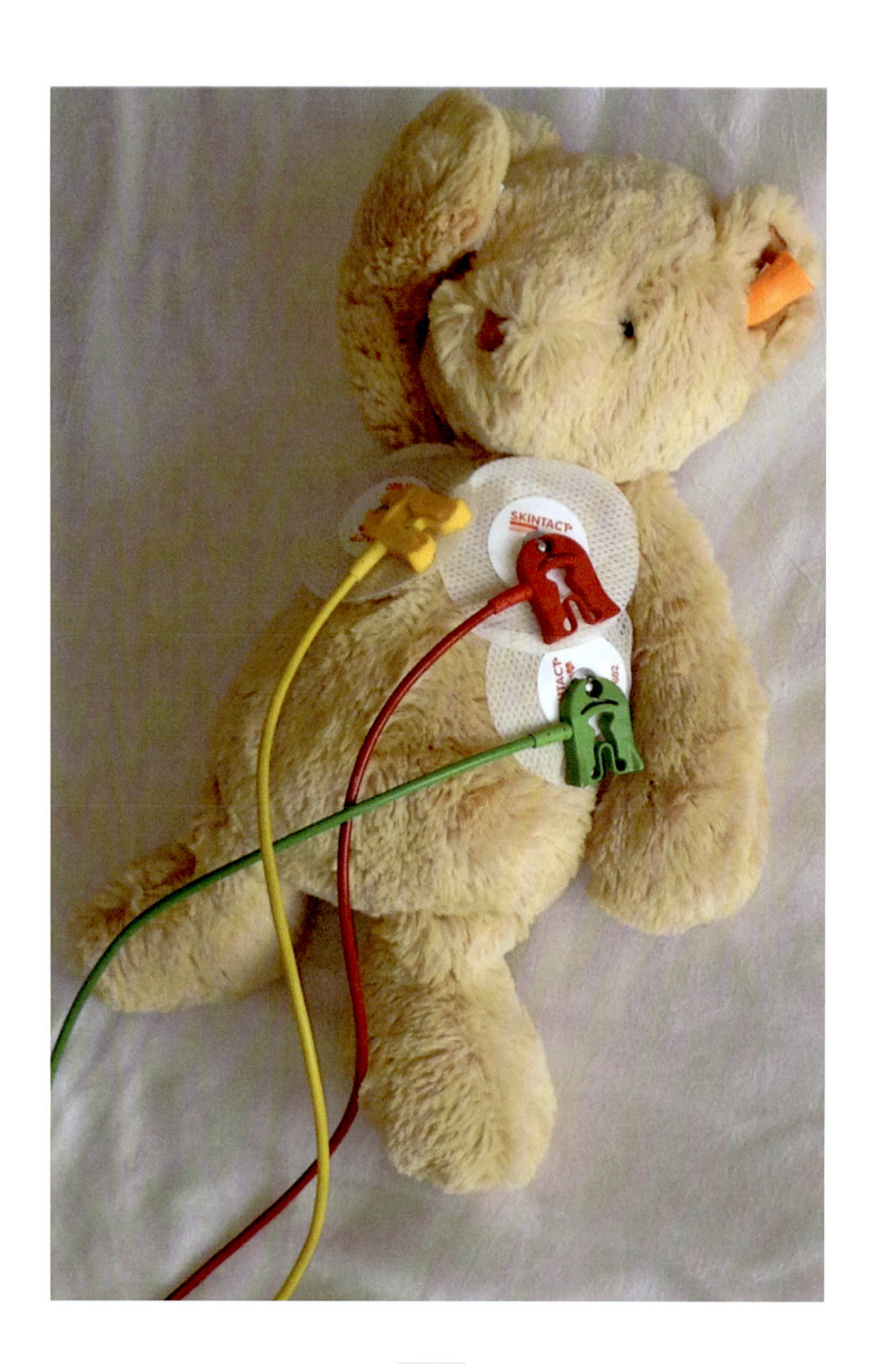

CHAPTER 5

"The very first requirement in a hospital is that it should do the sick no harm."

Florence Nightingale

As I travelled towards the hospital, my mobile phone rang, and the cardiologist's secretary asked for my ETA. She said that Dr. Schwarz was expecting me so they could start testing as soon as I arrived. As it happened, I was only a few minutes away and was pleased to see Rupert waiting for me at the entrance. We took the lift to the top floor and entered the High Dependency Unit. It felt like I was checking into a hotel as the reception area was stylised and did not look like a hospital at all.

'We have two rooms to offer you,' the receptionist said.

'Room 13 is the largest, but unfortunately the TV isn't working, and Room 12 is much smaller but with a functioning TV.'

'I'll take Room 12, thank you,' I said without hesitation and muttered to Rupert, 'I don't think I need any more bad luck.'

Rupert opened his eyes widely and grinned. We were then quickly escorted into a pleasant room which had a view of the City and a private bathroom. The rear wall had all the computer equipment, oxygen, and other paraphernalia of a high dependency room but the wall opposite the bed was decorated tastefully with a modern wallpaper and there was a leather sofa, coffee table and armchair by the window, which cleverly provided the patient with a normalised view whilst lying in bed. It turned out to be the right decision as I stayed in that cosy hospital room for 7 weeks while they tried to discover what was ailing me.

The cardiologist appeared invigorated at the thought of getting his teeth into such a 'fascinating' case. Rupert remarked that he sounded quite arrogant. He certainly seemed very serious and was a rather dour individual, but at this stage I didn't mind his shortcomings in this area if he found out what was going on and might get me better.

Rupert stayed for a little while and settled me in before going home, a two-hour journey ahead of him. The phlebotomist arrived and took multiple phials of blood, and one specialist after another filed into the room to take my medical history, hoping that one of their specialties would provide some clues. They attached me to a heart monitor which registered a resting pulse of 130bpm.

After a little while, Audette, the Head of Catering, came in with a menu and asked what I would like to eat for supper. She was a French lady, elegantly dressed, and was very knowledgeable about cuisine. I was quite surprised at how appetising the menu looked. The descriptions were more akin to a Michelin Star restaurant than the High Dependency Unit of a London hospital. The food arrived promptly and was delicious. It was reassuring to think that at least I would enjoy my meals there, even though I felt like a captive attached to electrical cables, my every move being monitored. Little did I know that eventually I would know the menu off by heart and would be allowed to request some favourite dishes as I stayed there so long.

I watched a little TV, but the audio was very distorted, and I couldn't concentrate as it sounded like the newsreader was underwater. I tried to settle on the rubber bed, but the cotton blankets weighed heavily and chafed as I strived to get warm. Luckily, I had brought my trusty foam pillow with me, and it provided a little home comfort. The air conditioning was particularly fierce and by midnight I was pacing the room in my coat and slippers moaning about the temperature, my fingers and toes as white as driven snow.

They're going to kill me in here, I ranted, the door of the staff room constantly squeaking outside in the corridor as they walked in and out, interspersed with alarm bells throughout the ward, machinery noises and my blood pressure cuff going off at regular intervals.

How is someone supposed to sleep in this inhospitable environment? I thought to myself.

I was grateful to have the room to myself but wasn't sure the arctic conditions would improve my well-being. I rang the bell for a nurse to see if they could turn down the air conditioning but was informed that the temperature was controlled centrally and not by individual room. Some extra cotton blankets were delivered but unfortunately in layers they became incredibly heavy and weren't particularly warm. One very helpful nurse went off to find some Elastoplast and taped over part of the a/c duct which made a huge difference and gradually the temperature increased. I suppose I was grumpy as I didn't want to be there, and this was my way of coping.

After an eventful night, I must have dozed off for a couple of hours and when I awoke it was around 5am. I grasped my smartphone which was on the bedside table and started to surf the internet to see if anything new might jump out and inspire me. I had been surfing every day since I was signed off work and my laptop grew hotter and hotter as the pressure to find a diagnosis continued. There were plenty of emails from the US to go through and then the end of shift nurse arrived to take my blood pressure reading.

The following day they provided me with a radiator, Luciana brought in some ear plugs and my parents came with a new duvet and bed socks. Finally, I would be able to get some well-earned rest. The catering staff entered my room at 8am and asked what I would like for breakfast. Again, the choice was amazing, and their culinary delights provided me with a small window of normality to the outside world. As I sat there munching my breakfast, I decided to turn on the TV and instead of watching the news found some cookery shows which helped to take my mind off my predicament. As it was a Saturday, nothing much was happening at the hospital. The tests would continue on Monday and so I spent the day getting dressed, receiving visitors, eating, watching TV, talking on the phone and surfing the internet. I didn't feel like reading the numerous books I had brought with me, which included the inauspiciously titled *The Woman who Went to Bed for a Year* by Sue Townsend. I figured it would be humorous and light, but I just couldn't settle my mind enough to read it.

I wasn't allowed to walk around the ward and had to stay in my room attached to the heart monitor. Obviously, this was completely foreign to me. Fortunately, my brain was still functioning, but I did not feel at all comfortable in this hostage situation and it had increased tenfold my usual hypervigilant state.

On Monday morning, the cardiologist arrived early and explained that he would be sending me by ambulance to two different hospitals for further tests. They came to collect me with a wheelchair, and I dressed up as though I was going to the Antarctic, with fur-lined boots, gloves, scarf, and a woolly hat. Despite feeling cold, I was perspiring, clammy across my abdomen and looked very grey.

The first test was a specialised MRI to measure the extent of inflammation in the heart, the second a PET CT scan to see if there was any evidence of the disease in the other internal organs. I had become accustomed to the MRI scanner, but the PET CT scan was very different. I had to lie still for an hour after they injected me with a radioactive sugar substance. It was all becoming very scary, and I looked forward to returning to the relative safety of my hospital bed. A nurse from the hospital had accompanied me in the ambulance and it took the best part of the day to complete. I wasn't allowed any food and by the end of the tests I was absolutely starving.

Audette, the Head of Catering, had come into my room several times during the day wondering where I was and luckily foresaw the need to make me a delicious dinner for my return to the ward. It's interesting how these little things can make such a difference. We had struck up an immediate friendship when I arrived as she was originally from Brittany, and it gave us both the opportunity to speak in French and take our minds off the seriousness of the situation.

The next day I felt rather optimistic and hoped that the tests might provide some clues as to what was going on with my little heart. The monitoring apparatus was still registering a resting heart rate of 105bpm and my blood pressure remained consistently low.

Dr. Schwarz walked into the room for an update. He sounded a little less sure of what was happening, the MRI and PET CT scan having provided very few clues. I was having regular troponin T and NT-proBNP blood tests which still looked as though I'd just suffered a massive heart attack.

'I'm afraid we're going to have to repeat all your entry blood tests... as the lab seems to have lost them,' he announced sheepishly.

I was already feeling like a pin cushion, and this was not welcome news. The monitor started to bleat like a lamb removed from its mother as I attempted to ask a few pertinent questions. The heart rate surged to 140bpm, and I started feeling clammy again. I decided to unplug the lead as the constant noise was so distracting and was making me feel even more distressed as I tried to field questions about the next steps. He told me he would review everything again after the results of the repeat blood tests.

I yearned for someone to give me some encouraging news. As he was leaving the room, he added.

'Your condition is very rare. We only usually see this at autopsy. You may eventually need a heart transplant.'

Well, that's encouraging! I thought to myself, as I leaned over to reattach the heart monitor.

Perhaps I should give him a pet name too... 'Dr. Doom', I decided, as he left the room like a black oil slick.

I couldn't help thinking that it is so important not to take away someone's hope; after all, it might be all they have.

I sat there for a moment staring out of the window and then turned on the TV to distract myself. Again, I didn't feel like watching the news. As I flicked through the channels, I found an old episode of *Everybody Loves Raymond*. The door opened and in came my breakfast. I started to chuckle and began to have belly laughs. After about half an hour I looked at the monitor as it had been unusually quiet. It registered 85bpm, 20 points lower than usual.

Could the comedy have had such a positive effect on me? I wondered.

I watched another episode, this time it was *Frasier*. Same effect, the monitor stayed at 85bpm. I finally got out of bed and unplugged the monitor to take a shower. I was trying to keep to a routine of showering, getting dressed and sitting in the chair, instead of lying in bed and becoming institutionalised. It was more and more burdensome to dry my hair as I found it difficult to hold my arms above my head for any length of time, and I had to sit down constantly.

Despite the sunny summer weather outside I often felt cold and was wearing socks, slippers, and warm clothing. Pulling the electric radiator towards me while sitting in the chair, I fired up my laptop and started surfing the internet, checking the symptoms of my condition, and answering the numerous emails from concerned friends and family. Knowledge was proving to be my ally against anxiety as I was becoming more and more skilful at navigating the numerous health websites and better at avoiding those which gave poor information. Of course, there were also those that tried to take advantage of sick people by forcing the purchase of an e-book to access the information about a particular illness, locking the computer into the site and only a reboot would close the connection.

The phlebotomist came in and took multiple phials of blood. I began to feel like I was taking part in an episode of *House*, except that there didn't seem to be a 'Dr. House' at this hospital, and no one had any clues as to what was ailing me.

One morning, I woke up with a start and for a split second wondered if it had all been a bad dream. I looked around the room and realised I was still in hospital, the reassuring beep of the heart monitor continued in the background. My heart was usually steady and fairly well-behaved after a night's sleep, although I couldn't say it was uninterrupted sleep as the squeaks of the staff room door continued incessantly throughout the night and the frequent visit of the night nurse to take my blood pressure would interrupt my fitful slumber. However, after a few weeks I had managed to negotiate an exception and avoid the 4am BP reading and they kindly agreed to make it 6am, which was a good compromise.

Luciana came in with my mail and a change of clothes every few days. She even brought in an aerosol can of lubricating oil and I managed to get one of the helpful catering staff to spray it on the hinges of the staff room door to allay the squeaking. After lunch, I felt the need to distract myself. I was able to enjoy movies and TV programmes but didn't feel comfortable reading anything apart from research. My brain was just racing too much. I took out several DVDs and found *The House of Cards*, the original version with Ian Richardson, which Maria had given me during her visit at the weekend. I put the first DVD into the side of the TV and pressed play on the remote. Although it was set in Westminster, it reminded me of some of the unfortunate characters I had met in my working life. I ended up watching numerous episodes in one go. It was wonderfully distracting.

I felt a shudder as I received a call from one of those very colleagues, just as I was watching the programme. Pandora announced that she wanted to come and see me and no doubt report back to Nigel. She had a fearsome reputation of being the office henchman and one to whom unpopular tasks would be delegated. I felt a little anxious at the thought of her visit and wasn't sure what to expect. However, I was hoping the severity of my condition might induce a modicum of compassion, although I'd never observed it in the past. I put it out of my mind for the moment and concentrated on replying to emails. Another couple of visitors turned up and the time flew by. I had an ever-increasing number of get well cards displayed on the wall opposite my bed as well as flowers and balloons which were quite heartening.

One evening, I called Virginia to see how she was doing. Virginia has been a close friend for many years, and we have been on many hilarious adventures together in the past. On one holiday, we went to stay at a medieval house near Carcassonne, which an erstwhile boyfriend of Virginia's had just bought. We rented a small car at the airport and on the Sunday morning drove to the house near a small village called Limoux in southwest France. The weather had been very wet, and as we drove into the property, the custodian was waiting to meet us. He gave us a tour and as we walked into the house Virginia and I both felt a strange sense of foreboding. There was an array of unfinished construction work throughout, and we found two bedrooms at the top, one with an enormous 7ft bed. As there was no food in the house, we decided to go out for a drive and find a supermarket or restaurant. It was too late for lunch so we walked around the town and checked out a hotel where we might stay as alternative accommodation, but as there was no access by car, we decided it would be impractical.

Upon returning to Limoux, we found a quaint family restaurant to have dinner, savouring their sparkling wine, Crémant de Limoux, which was light, bubbly, and delicious. It is said that the monks of Saint Hilaire Abbey near Limoux perfected the winemaking method for sparkling wines around 1531. When the infamous Dom Pérignon made a pilgrimage to Saint Hilaire Abbey, he was taught the method and used the technique on Champagne wines when he returned to Hautvillers Abbey. Hence the Champagne method was learned from the monks in Limoux.

On the way back to the house, we stopped off at a corner shop to purchase some milk, ham, and eggs for breakfast. As we walked back to the car, we suddenly felt enormous raindrops falling out of the menacing sky. Virginia drove off at speed, the driving rain swept aside by the squeaking windscreen wipers. It was very dark, with no streetlights whatsoever and as we mounted the hill to the house above, we could feel a storm brewing and the wind was gathering speed. As I exited the car to find the key that was hidden on a little ledge in the barn, I was buffeted by the wind and quickly became wet in the driving rain. We unloaded the suitcases from the car and went inside. The house was very dimly lit, and I went upstairs to the bathroom on the first floor. The door to the bathroom was very old, covered in woodworm with a rusty bolt fastening. As I pushed the door open, I stopped in my tracks as there were small granules of glass spread all over the bathroom floor. It looked like the shower screen over the bath had exploded. Thinking we had left a window open, I checked but the latch was firmly fastened. It made absolutely no sense at all as we hadn't even used the bathroom. At this point I called out to Virginia who was in the kitchen making us some camomile tea.

'Quick, come and look at this,' I said

Virginia mounted the stairs at speed and entered the bathroom. The shattered glass was everywhere.

'How strange that the hinge is just sitting perfectly on the edge of the bath' she said, 'almost as though someone has placed it there.'

We went to find a dustpan and brush and spent the next hour scooping the glass into the bath. We left the suitcases downstairs, just taking out the items that we needed overnight. As we went back upstairs, we both decided to stay in the same room with the gigantic bed as neither of us felt particularly safe and secure. Virginia was the first to go off to sleep and I lay there on my back feeling on edge and unable to relax. I kept getting up to go to the bathroom and noticed that around forty centipedes were now crawling all over the broken glass in the bath. As I climbed back into bed, Virginia stirred and said,

'You don't seem very settled'.

'Settled!' I said incredulously. 'I've just scratched my arm on that rusty door, I've probably now got tetanus!'

The wind was howling outside, and the rain was lashing at the windows. Virginia picked up a *Reader's Digest* which was on her bedside table and gave it to me with a little purple book light, although the mount was broken, and I had to keep swinging it around to illuminate the page. It was a special edition to commemorate the anniversary of 9/11, hardly appropriate reading in the circumstances. Suddenly, there was an almighty crash downstairs,

'Did you hear that?' I said to Virginia. It sounded as though someone had thrown a chair across the living room. We both lay hiding under the sheet, wondering what was happening.

I stayed there not moving for quite a while and then heard Virginia's breathing change which gave the impression that she had gone back to sleep. After a short while, I began to hear the soft murmuring of voices downstairs. A man and a woman were talking but I couldn't hear what was being said as it was too far away. I didn't say anything to Virginia as she was sleeping soundly, and I wasn't sure if I was imagining it. I stayed awake all night until the storm broke and the sun was beginning to rise. At this point, I dropped off to sleep for a few hours and awoke again around 8am. Virginia was also stirring beside me.

'Virginia, we're going to a hotel,' I announced firmly as I jumped out of bed to find my robe. 'There's no way I'm staying here any longer,' I continued. 'Did you hear those noises in the night?'

'Yes,' Virginia concurred, 'and what about those voices?'

'That's it,' I said, 'the place must be haunted! Let's get dressed, have breakfast and get out of here.'

Virginia went downstairs to make breakfast while I had a shower, got dressed and rang a travel agent to try and find alternative accommodation. Unfortunately, what Virginia had bought for breakfast turned out to be raw bacon instead of ham, so we decided to give breakfast a miss. As Virginia ventured outside, she discovered the rear door of the rental car was wide open and the rain had made the seat all wet.

'I'm sure I locked the car when we came in last night,' she said furrowing her brow.

'I think the sooner we get out of here the better,' I replied.

As we drove away from the house of horrors, we called the custodian to let him know we would be leaving early.

'Anything wrong?' he asked before Virginia told him the story of the exploding shower screen.

'We think it might be haunted also,' she continued.

'Funny you should say that, but none of the builders like working there,' he said.

We drove away quickly to a hotel by the sea and finally managed to enjoy our holiday.

Getting back to the hospital, I had just ordered some hot chocolate and was munching on a delicious bar of milk chocolate that Virginia had given me a couple of days beforehand, while speaking to her on the phone. Virginia was in a bit of a state and was having serious problems at work. As I tried to offer support, the heart monitor started to bleep very loudly, and the heart rate had increased significantly. It appeared the mixture of the chocolate and the stress was impacting my heart. As the nurse came in to see what was happening, she mentioned that her husband had experienced a similar reaction to chocolate and that perhaps it was the theobromine content which might have been stimulating my heart. Apparently, that's the ingredient in chocolate that kills dogs. Every time I tried to eat chocolate the same thing happened. It would be three years before I could safely eat it again.

Most days I had a visitor around 7pm and we often ate dinner together which helped to keep me sane. Audette provided me with the most delicious meals and she and her staff were a positive complement to my treatment. It was as though they were nourishing me, not only with their delicious and wholesome food, but also their kindness, care and attention and I mopped it up like a sponge. On one occasion Rupert came to see me and my heart skipped a beat as he entered the room. Of course, missed beats were the norm for me at this point but he dined out on that story for weeks afterwards.

Pandora sashayed unannounced into my room one morning as I was having my daily blood pressure check. She had brought a box of Belgian seashell chocolates with her. I didn't like to say I would not be able to eat them, but they turned out to be a delicious treat for my other visitors. I continued to look exceedingly pale with a greyish tinge, and rather disturbingly my knees had taken on a bluish hue. My ability to walk had slowed considerably and any exertion whatsoever rendered me short of breath. I suppose Pandora took one look at me and decided to back off. The monitor was firmly attached and would bleat occasionally during her visit providing a reassuring defence. After about 15 minutes another nurse came in to conduct further tests and Pandora was asked to wait outside.

I was incredibly relieved when Joaquin arrived, and Pandora took the cue to leave. He looked relaxed and was wearing a Mickey Mouse T-shirt. His curly brown hair had flecks of grey and it was surprising that he could get away with such a fashion statement, but he was one of those people who would look good wearing just a paper bag.

'Who was that?' he asked as he passed Pandora on her way out.

'Oh, that's Pandora from work,' I replied.

'What's she like?' He asked.

I smiled and said, 'A chocolate-covered spider.' We both giggled mischievously.

Joaquin made himself comfortable on the sofa and we talked about his wedding plans. It was good to talk about something other than my health. The civil ceremony was going to take place in Milan in a few weeks, but they were planning a huge event later in the year in Argentina and he insisted that I get better so that I could attend.

After Joaquin had left, I started contemplating a trip to Argentina to attend the wedding and decided to make it one of my goals. As I sat there dreaming, I took a pen and a sheet of paper to write a list of things I would like to do:

When I get better...

1. Attend Joaquin's Wedding in Argentina
2. Learn how to dance the Tango in Buenos Aires
3. Write my book
4. Learn how to speak Spanish
5. Start painting again
6. Visit Tuscany and do a cookery course
7. Visit Rome and Florence
8. Go to the Chassagne Montrachet wine region
9. Watch Roger Federer play tennis at Wimbledon
10. Swim in the sea
11. Eat a meal cooked by James Martin or Raymond Blanc
12. Live somewhere with warm weather

My Results

Ejection Fraction: 32%
Cardiac High Sensitivity Troponin T: 110 ng/L
BNP (NT-proBNP): 8500 ng/L

CHAPTER 6

"The art of life lies in a constant readjustment to our surroundings."

Okakura Kakuzo

As the weeks passed, I continued to have endless examinations, tests, echos, and MRIs, but nothing provided a definitive diagnosis. At this point I was starting to lose hope that they would find out what was wrong with me before I succumbed to the inevitable. They tried out various medications, including beta blockers and ACE inhibitors, but they turned me into a sloth, unable to function and the beta blockers were provoking Raynaud's in the middle of the night. Nothing seemed to help, and they were fast running out of ideas.

Whilst researching, I saw an article in the health section of the daily newspaper featuring 'broken heart syndrome'. It is medically known as 'takotsubo cardiomyopathy' and sometimes known as 'stress cardiomyopathy'. The word 'takotsubo' originates from the word for a Japanese octopus trap, as the left ventricle of the heart changes into a similar shape to the trap, developing a narrow neck and a round bottom. This condition provokes a sudden temporary weakening of the muscular portion of the heart and usually appears suddenly after a significant stressor, either physical or emotional, hence the term 'broken heart'. I began to wonder if all that insidious stress at work had taken its toll. However, I didn't have the archetypal 'takotsubo' shape of the left ventricle, which is unique to this condition, although I couldn't help thinking that all the relentless pressure had been deleterious to my heart.

Over the last month, in my various discussions with Dr. Schwarz, he mentioned that if we had made no further progress that he would have to perform a myocardial biopsy. I was not looking forward to that procedure. The idea of taking several small pieces of my heart filled me with dread.

Later that day Virginia came to have dinner with me and brought a bunch of flowers. She tended to them and then came and sat on my bed. I no longer had any colour in my cheeks and felt more comfortable lying down than sitting in the chair. I suppose the last four weeks had caught up with me and I was concerned about the myocardial biopsy which was looming.

Virginia's effervescence was somewhat diminished also that evening. I put it down to problems she was having at work, but it turned out that she was beginning to wonder if I was going to make it. Of course, she didn't say anything to me at the time, only to tell me at a future date, but gave me a huge hug before she left, which was somewhat out of character.

As Virginia was leaving, Joaquin arrived and although I felt tired, I didn't want to discourage him from visiting me. He looked a little sad and mentioned that his favourite horse, Ximena, had just died of a heart attack.

'Well, I have no intention of going anywhere,' I said reassuringly, trying to conceal my extreme exhaustion.

After we talked about what had happened to Ximena, I asked,

'Do you believe in God Joaquin?'

Joaquin pondered briefly and replied

'I do with my heart but not with my head.'

I reflected on what he had said as he gazed at me tenderly. Then suddenly he detected a change in atmosphere.

'Are you OK Dino?' he asked all at once looking concerned. 'Dino, Dino, Dino,' he repeated, his soft brown eyes locked onto mine.

'Yes, I'm fine,' I fibbed, hoping he wouldn't notice. 'Just a bit tired.'

I tried to reassure him that it was nothing and that I would be OK. He hesitated for a while, not wanting to leave, but I told him again not to worry. He hugged me tightly as though he didn't want to release me too quickly and then left.

As I stayed there alone, I realised the graveness of my predicament. I had been desperately trying to find a solution, but every avenue led to a dead end. I was starting to feel frantic that we would run out of time and maybe that's what Joaquin had detected. John, the nurse who was taking care of the night shift, came in to check on me. He asked me who my visitor was and mentioned that he had often seen him arriving late in the evening to visit me. I told him about Joaquin, how kind he was and how very sad I felt that he had lost his favourite horse.

'People who like animals are often very kind,' he said.

'Yes, I guess you're right. I've never really thought about it that way,' I replied.

'You're so brave,' he said.

I paused for a moment and then replied.

'Well, you know you can only be brave if you feel frightened.'

John left the room and I settled under my duvet. I slept well but was awoken early by a team of nurses who were preparing me for the myocardial biopsy. I was so glad they hadn't told me the day before as I would not have slept a wink all night worrying about it.

A seasoned Irish nurse, Bernadette, was going to accompany me to the surgical floor and return with me to my room afterwards. I called my friend Clare and asked if she could come to the hospital for my return to the ward. As luck would have it, she answered the phone immediately and came straight from home. It would take her an hour to travel across London. I called my parents to let them know also. The team came in and I was transferred to another bed to be wheeled downstairs. As we arrived on the surgical ward, I noticed that twenty beds were lined up with patients, each waiting to enter theatre. It felt like being on a conveyor belt. Bernadette was reassuring and I was so glad she was with me.

Dr. Schwarz was waiting for me as they wheeled me into the operating room. Everything looked icy blue and, as they transferred me onto the cold metal table, they covered me in a silver foil space blanket. The trepidation was palpable. My heart rate was elevated, and I was given a sedative to keep me calm. After disinfecting the area, Dr. Schwarz introduced a sheath into the vein in my groin and inserted the bioptome, threading it towards the right ventricle with the aid of a special type of moving X-ray called fluoroscopy.

As it reached the right ventricle, I felt several ectopic beats. The instrument felt as though it was tickling my heart and irritating it. I informed Dr. Schwarz and he administered a bit more sedative. I could see everything happening on the screen beside me. Carefully he positioned the bioptome to extract the first biopsy. He then repositioned it to extract another piece from a different side of the right ventricle. Just one more piece to take and then we would be finished. The last piece took a little longer. As he drew out the catheter, I felt such a sense of relief. Pressure was applied to the wound in my groin to stop the bleeding.

He had placed all the pieces into a container with a preservative and asked me to make sure I knew where it was. I kept my eyes firmly on that biopsy, fretting that it would be mislaid, like my first blood tests, and I would have to go through the procedure all over again. I was particularly concerned as it was a Friday, and the following Monday was the summer bank holiday. Finally, a nurse called Linda came to retrieve the biopsy and wandered out of the room. Dr. Schwarz came back into the operating theatre to collect it and asked me where it had gone. I pointed him in the direction of the nurse who had taken it and gave him her name. I was transferred to a holding bay and my friendly nurse, Bernadette, was there smiling. Dr. Doom walked past holding the container and for the first time appeared to be smiling too.

By 11am I returned to the ward and Clare was there waiting for me. It was so great to see her.

'Hello Baby, how was it?' she asked, looking optimistic.

'Well, actually, it wasn't as bad as I thought Clare. The only bit that was disconcerting was when the probe was irritating my heart, but luckily that didn't last too long,' I replied reassuringly.

'When will you get the results?' she added

'I'm not too sure, I will have to check.' I managed to get up and go to the bathroom, with my leg outstretched and we spent a pleasant afternoon together.

My parents had driven up from the country and were staying in my flat for the weekend so that they would be able to come and visit me. Maria was also planning to come to the hospital.

The following morning, as Maria arrived, I was

watching *Saturday Kitchen* with the lovely James Martin. We watched it together for a while. Maria loved food and was married to a chef. I gave her back the box set of *The House of Cards*.

'Isn't it amazing?' she said. 'It reminds me so much of Nigel!'

'I know!' I continued, 'I'm so glad I'm not having to cope with that at the moment.'

'Have you heard from him?' she added

'No, not a word! Just from Pandora, but no doubt she has reported back.'

It crossed my mind that Nigel was probably disappointed I hadn't yet succumbed to the inevitable. I'd occasionally observed him appear to relish the misfortune of others and to enjoy the drama of it all, almost in a macabre way. Unfortunately, there even exists a German word for that – 'Schadenfreude'.

At that point, my parents arrived, and I ordered tea and coffee for everyone. They already knew Maria very well as we had been friends since our early twenties. We looked at the lunch menu and Maria asked my father, who had become rather hard of hearing,

'Do you like moussaka?'

'No starter for me,' he replied breezily.

'No, I didn't actually say that,' Maria continued and repeated a little louder,

'Do you like moussaka?'

'Who's she?' he said.

We all burst out laughing. It was good to have something to lighten the mood. After lunch, my father, who enjoys photography, took some pictures and then Maria decided it was time for her to go home.

As she hugged me goodbye, she started to cry. I was

quite taken aback as Maria had always been quite stoic. I looked around the room and my father had taken out his handkerchief and was wiping back a tear too. As I turned to my mother, I could see her eyes welling up also. The atmosphere was suddenly laden with emotion too painful to articulate.

Oh dear, I thought as I could feel a lump rising in my throat.

'Come on Maria, I'll be alright,' I said, giving her a big hug and trying to defuse the emotional storm that was fast erupting. Everyone had been so strong up to that point. I wasn't sure I could cope with anything else.

After Maria left, my parents stayed another couple of hours. We watched the movie that Maria had brought with her, *Something's Gotta Give*, which was excellent and then they left the hospital to go back to my apartment.

As my parents stood on the side of the street hailing a cab, someone pushed in front of them. The taxi driver drove around the interloper and stopped in front of my mother.

'Ah that's kind of you,' she said, 'I thought we had lost you.'

'No, no,' exclaimed the driver, 'I saw you were waiting before that other chap. Please get in.'

As my parents took their seats in the back and gave the address, the driver started chatting to them.

'Have you just been to the hospital?' he asked.

'Yes, we've just been to visit our daughter,' my mother replied

'What's she in for?' he continued

'Well, it's something to do with her heart. She's been there a month already and they don't know what's wrong.'

'I'm sorry to hear that,' he said.

They continued chatting about other things and arrived in front of my building in no time. As my mother exited the cab and stood in front of the window to pay, the driver asked,

'What's your daughter's name?'
'It's Kayte,' she said.
'Kayte with a "Y"' he replied.
'YES!' she said, amazed that he would know that.
'She will be alright; I will pray for her,' he replied.
My mother could feel the hairs on her arms stand on end.
'Thank you very much,' she said as they said goodbye.

As soon as they were safely in the apartment, she called me to recount the story. I too felt goosebumps as she told me what he had said.

My Results

Ejection Fraction: 28%
Cardiac High Sensitivity Troponin T: 131 ng/L
BNP (NT-proBNP): 6020 ng/L

CHAPTER 7

"When you have exhausted all the possibilities, remember this; you haven't."

Thomas Edison

As I waited for the results of the biopsy, the days went past and I spent the time again receiving visitors, watching movies, and doing research on my laptop. One morning at about 7.30am I was sleeping on my front and was awoken by a professor beside my bed clicking his heels so loudly that it sounded like a rifle had been fired. I quickly turned over and saw a tall, slim man with glasses. He leaned forward to shake my hand and I noted that it felt rather moist. I asked him to take a seat, always mindful of my NLP training, and he obliged, sat down and made his declaration.

'You have undifferentiated connective tissue disease.'

I was quite taken aback as I thought my diagnosis was still unknown and I was still awaiting the results of the biopsy.

'Is that the same as mixed connective tissue disease?' I asked.

'Ah my students often make that mistake,' he continued. 'No, it's different,' and went on to explain what it was.

'I will write on your notes the treatment I would recommend in your case,' he said confidently.

His mind was obviously made up and I couldn't understand why I had been lying there for four weeks if it were that obvious and, up to now, I'd had no treatment. I had done some reading on connective tissue disorders when they had first mentioned scleroderma and in particular some research that was being carried out in Germany. I mentioned this to him, but he replied quite indignantly,

'I'm not interested in what goes on in the rest of Europe, I'm only interested in what's happening in the UK.'

I couldn't quite believe my ears. Here was someone entering my hospital room, waking me up, giving me his diagnosis, presenting me with his viewpoint and not considering any work done elsewhere. I bit my tongue, but the monitor decided to bleep loudly instead of me and again I had to unplug it. I must say the whole episode did not improve my mood.

Later that day, my spirits rose as Sharon came to visit with her little boy Henry. He was only four years old but was extremely well-behaved and his mother had warned him to expect lots of machines. Henry came in holding a glorious posy of summer flowers and placed it on my bed.

'Oh, thank you Henry,' I said smiling at him. 'They're gorgeous!'

He looked very pleased with himself and went and sat down on a chair in the corner in a determined fashion.

'Would you like something to drink Henry?' I asked.

'Yeth please,' he said softly.

We ordered some tea and an orange juice for Henry.

As Sharon handed the glass to him, it appeared enormous within his tiny frame. His hands were trembling as he lifted the glass to his lips, desperately trying not to spill it on his school uniform. He was wearing an oversized charcoal grey blazer with a wire embroidered badge on the chest pocket.

How darling, I thought as I looked at him. It was a joy to be distracted by such a delightful little boy, blissfully unaware of what was going on around him.

I slept quite well that night and awoke as usual around 6am on Friday morning. The nurse who took my first blood pressure of the day had not yet done his rounds. I started to look at my smartphone again. Having done quite a lot of research, I kept coming across the term 'myocarditis'. I had many of the symptoms and wondered if I might be on the right track. After my usual morning routine, I spoke to my mother on the phone around 11am.

'I think I've got myocarditis,' I said

'Why do you think that?' she replied

'I can't see what else it can be, nothing else seems to fit.'

On Friday evening, around 6pm Dr. Schwarz charged into my room.

'We've got your diagnosis from the cardiac biopsy,' he said breezily.

'What is it?' I asked in anticipation.

'It's myocarditis,' he said, relieved that finally he had the answer.

'I will come and talk to you on Monday about what we plan to do.'

I rang my mother straight away to tell her.

'It's myocarditis!'

'That's what you said this morning,' she replied.

'I know!' I said feeling somewhat vindicated.

The following day, armed with my diagnosis, I began to surf the internet to find out all I could about myocarditis. I looked on YouTube and found a video featuring a man called Dr. Leslie Cooper who was based at the Mayo Clinic and who appeared to be an authority on the disease. I looked up the phone number of the clinic and called immediately.

A security guard answered the phone. He was very friendly and informed me that the clinic was closed until Monday and that I should call back then. I checked the time. They were six hours behind. He gave me the direct number of Dr. Cooper's office and I made a note of it. During my research I had also found a very interesting medical publication called *Progress in Cardiovascular Diseases*. It was written by Lori A. Blauwet and Leslie T. Cooper. It contained an excellent chapter on myocarditis and I felt like I might be making some progress, at last.

The rest of the weekend was spent receiving visitors and passing the time in the usual way but I felt quite excited at the prospect of being able to speak to Dr. Cooper on Monday. As I was now on my fifth week, I was impatient to do something finally that might make a difference.

Early on Monday morning Dr. Doom entered my room purposefully.

'We're going to give you lots of nasty drugs now,' he announced abruptly.

Buoyed with the knowledge that I would be speaking to an expert later that day, I felt confident to take control of my situation.

'Well firstly I'd like to know what medication you plan to give me and secondly I'd like a second opinion,' I said in a determined fashion. He looked at me rather startled, going quite scarlet around the gills.

'Well, you haven't known what to do for five weeks so I think I'm entitled to a second opinion from someone who is an expert in this disease. I have waited this long I really don't see how another day is going to make very much difference,' I said firmly.

Dr. Schwarz left the room somewhat deflated, but I was determined to proceed along this path. I had always believed it was respectful to apply the appropriate deference to the clinician, but now I felt like I needed to regain some important control over my life. I kept looking at my watch, but I couldn't call until 3pm, which would have been 9am US time. When the time finally arrived, I called the number and managed to get straight through. Dr. Cooper's secretary answered,

'Dr. Cooper's office.' she said brightly.

'Hello,' I said, 'I've just been diagnosed with myocarditis, I am currently in hospital and was wondering if I might speak to Dr. Cooper. I'm willing to pay for the consultation.'

'Ah my dear, I think he might be in the exercise room with a patient, let me see if I can put you through,' she replied helpfully.

I was so relieved to make contact, never thinking that it would be that simple. It had been very difficult to talk to anyone in the UK about my condition without going through the formal channels. After a couple of minutes Dr. Cooper came on the line. He was incredibly friendly and was willing to answer a whole host of questions that I had prepared for him. It was evident that he knew so much about myocarditis. We talked about whom I might consult in London, and he gave me a few names. We also talked about the treatments available for my condition. I told him that they had experienced a great deal of difficulty getting me on the heart medication, and he suggested that a way to approach it would be titration, administering small quantities of a drug and gradually building up slowly until the body adapted to it.

We must have been on the phone for at least half an hour and when I put down the receiver I felt totally uplifted. The heavy black cloud had started to rise, and I finally felt I might be making some progress.

I called my parents to tell them the good news.

'I want to check out of the hospital and go to America to see Dr. Cooper,' I said with a newfound vigour in my voice.

My father thought that perhaps it wasn't a good idea right now, but that I should go when I felt a bit stronger. Of course, he was right, there was no way I would have survived a flight in my current condition. My last echo had registered an ejection fraction of 28% and my heart was still severely inflamed.

Joaquin called later that morning and gave me the name of an Argentinian cardiologist based in London, who had been recommended by Dr. Love, his cardiologist friend in Argentina. I rang him immediately and he gave me the name of Professor White, who specialised in heart failure, together with his mobile telephone number. Interestingly, it happened to be one of the cardiologists whom Dr. Cooper had also recommended. When Dr. Schwarz came into my room that evening he gave me the name of my second opinion. It turned out to be the very same professor that all the others had mentioned, Professor White. All paths were now pointing in the same direction. It was finally coming together.

That evening, I texted Professor White and explained my situation. He had been to the theatre and rang me on his way home. He was incredibly friendly and sounded very reassuring.

'I will receive your notes and scans tomorrow and will call you when I have some news. In the meantime, try not to worry,' he said reassuringly.

Concurrently, my biopsy had been sent to various experts at two different hospitals to give their opinion on what might be the cause of the myocardial fibrosis. Then one morning Dr. Schwarz came into my room to report that one of my biopsies had been lost in the post.

'Why would anyone put my heart biopsy in the mail?' I asked, not quite believing how that had happened.

'If I had known they were going to do that I would've paid to put it in a black cab,' I continued in a tone of controlled exasperation, steam starting to escape from my ears.

He had no answers to give me and just shrugged his shoulders as he left. The monitor started to bleep madly again as I felt the stress and frustration rising. Unfortunately, when the other piece of heart tissue finally turned up in the mail, they were unable to extract any RNA because it had been stored incorrectly and the piece was too small. There was now no way of knowing if the myocarditis had been triggered by a virus or bacteria.

Despite all the challenges of that day, I managed to sleep well and hoped the following day might bring some positive news. Midway through the next morning I received a call from Professor White. He said that he had looked at my scans but unfortunately the disease was now across both left and right ventricles and that the only treatment option open to me was steroids and immunosuppressant drugs. However, he thought we should wait until the results of the biopsy to rule out any infection.

I then had to tell him the bad news that they had lost my biopsy in the mail and when it had finally turned up it couldn't be read as it hadn't been stored correctly. I thanked him for his help and asked if there were any possibility when I came out of hospital that I could transfer my care to him. He said that I would need permission from my current cardiologist, but he was happy to take me as a patient if he agreed.

After the phone call I sat there contemplating the prospect of taking high-dose steroids. I had very little experience of them but what I did know made me feel very concerned. For a while the room was empty and quiet. I could feel the tears welling up as I contemplated my future, the prospect of a long life ever more remote. I tried with all my might but finally an enormous tear plopped defiantly onto my cheek. Just at that moment Dr. Doom came into the room.

'What's wrong? Did the Professor tell you something you didn't want to hear?' he said in lofty scorn.

I couldn't quite believe the lack of empathy I was experiencing from this man particularly as there had been such a litany of errors throughout my hospital stay. I quickly steeled myself and with a surge of defiance asked him what he was proposing as a treatment. He replied that he was planning to put me on 3000mg of Solu-Medrol for three days and that it would be given intravenously.

After he left the room, I sat there deep in thought. Gradually my gaze fixed upon a little teddy bear that one of my friends, Alma, had given me a few days earlier. He was sitting in the window and looked rather forlorn. I walked over to rescue him and put him in my bed. It's funny how teddies bring reassurance when you're feeling vulnerable and frightened.

I couldn't sleep that night thinking about the Solu-Medrol treatment that was looming. I did a lot of research about it and finally watched a girl on YouTube who provided her own experience of the drug and said that your heart would beat out of your chest and that your skin would break down at the injection site. There were other serious side effects that she listed and, consequently, I didn't feel comfortable with the prospect of this treatment. I was certainly not convinced that beating my heart out of its chest was going to be helpful to me when it was doing that all on its own. This treatment seemed very extreme, and I wasn't convinced it was the right solution for me. What was the point of merely staying alive regardless of the quality of life?

At around 5am I woke up and said out loud

'I'm not going to do it!' 'And if they try and force me, I'm going to leave the hospital.'

My subconscious had decided this was not the right path and I would not be deflected.

A little later that morning, Serena called me to see how everything was going and asked whether I had started the steroids yet.

'No, they want to give me 3000mg of Solu-Medrol intravenously. I'm just not going to do it.'

'Goodness, that seems excessive,' she said reassuringly.

Fortunately, common sense prevailed and later that morning Dr. Schwarz informed me that after discussing the matter with other colleagues, he had decided to change the treatment to a much smaller dose of prednisolone and in pill form. I therefore no longer had to make my case against it.

As the days went by, Dr. Schwarz discussed the possibility of my having an ICD, an internal defibrillator which would be inserted in the heart in case I had a sudden cardiac arrest. I asked him a few questions about it.

'How many of these devices have you used for similar conditions?'

'Ten,' he replied.

'And how many have gone off,' I continued.

'Just the one,' he said.

My mind wandered off and I started to think about the movie *Manon des Sources*. There is a scene where Ugolin (who had become obsessed with Manon) takes a large needle and sews Manon's ribbon into his heart. As the film develops, the wound festers and eventually brings about his demise.

I couldn't imagine that it would be a good idea for my little heart to have the intrusion of a permanent foreign object, particularly as it had reacted so immediately to the bioptome during the cardiac biopsy. I was certainly not keen on having my body integrity assaulted. Thus, I decided that the risk–benefit ratio was not in my favour and placated Dr. Doom by saying I would think about it.

Later that day an electrophysiologist came into my room to discuss the benefits of the ICD and to encourage me to have one fitted. They certainly were persistent, but words of caution rarely slow the rush to treatment.

'It's not that you could have just a cardiac arrest,' he said alarmingly, 'you could have a stroke as well.'

'Oh well, I think I'll take my chances,' I said, starting to rebel against the medical establishment. At this point, I just wanted to go home. Perhaps I had a romantic idea of the strength of my own heart, but I was rejecting the prospect of a physically painful and dispiriting reminder of my mortality that I would be able to see and feel every day.

I decided to call Dr. Cooper again to ask his advice. I mentioned that they wanted to operate and insert an ICD, and I was concerned about it as my heart was already inflamed and it meant that I would not be able to have any further MRIs.

'There is an alternative that we use here in the States,' he said, offering a ray of hope. 'We sometimes use a "Zoll LifeVest." You wear it externally and when your heart improves you can take it off again.'

That felt like a very sensible solution, and someone was finally talking about my getting better. I checked YouTube and found a video explanation. It looked like a life jacket with a control pack which resembled a transistor radio. (See page 85.)

What Is the LifeVest Wearable Defibrillator?

The LifeVest™ wearable defibrillator is a treatment option for sudden cardiac arrest that offers patients advanced protection and monitoring as well as improved quality of life. Unlike an implantable cardioverter defibrillator (ICD), the LifeVest is worn outside the body rather than implanted in the chest. This device continuously monitors the patient's heart with dry, non-adhesive sensing electrodes to detect life-threatening abnormal heart rhythms. If a life-threatening rhythm is detected, the device alerts the patient prior to delivering a treatment shock, and thus allows a conscious patient to delay the treatment shock. If the patient becomes unconscious, the device releases a Blue™ gel over the therapy electrodes and delivers an electrical shock to restore normal rhythm.

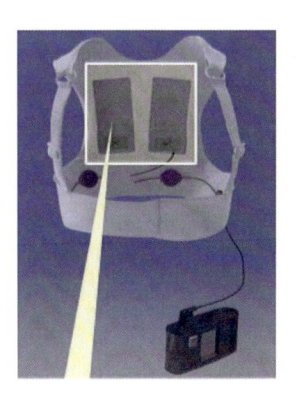

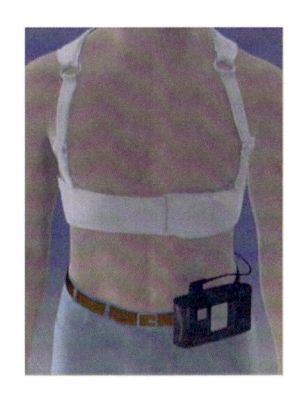

In the event of a life-threatening arrhythmia, these dry therapeutic electrodes will automatically deploy conductive gel prior to delivering a shock.

When Dr. Schwarz entered my room again, I told him that rather than an ICD, I would prefer to use a 'LifeVest'.

'What's that?' he asked, looking rather irritated. 'There's a lot of rubbish on the internet, you know!'

I took out my trusty smartphone again and played the video for him.

'I'll look into it and get back to you,' he said as he departed quickly, looking rather annoyed.

As my care was being transferred to Professor White, and my release date was looming, I had to start walking around the ward with a nurse so that I would be in a fit state to leave the hospital. I felt very unsteady on my legs and could not walk very fast. My ejection fraction was still very low and despite my feistiness I was not a well girl. In the end they still hadn't given me the steroid treatment because it was not clear if I might still have a virus or a bacterial infection because of the mismanagement of my cardiac biopsy. I had also asked Dr. Schwarz if he would be willing to test my vitamin D levels before I left. I had been reading quite a lot of research on the benefits of supplementation and it turned out I was severely deficient.

As I climbed into my parents' car on the day of my discharge, the enormity of what I had been through weighed heavily. I felt free at last, but incredibly weak and fragile. My mother had to drive very slowly as every bump in the road bothered my heart.

My Results

Ejection Fraction: 28%
Cardiac High Sensitivity Troponin T: 75 ng/L
BNP (NT-proBNP): 5150 ng/L
25-Hydroxy Vitamin D: 20nmol/L

CHAPTER 8

"The words of kindness are more healing to a drooping heart than balm or honey."

Sarah Fielding

As I finally lay in my own bed that night, I suddenly felt very vulnerable. I had been attached to a heart monitor for seven weeks and now I no longer had the reassurance that if something untoward should happen that a nurse would come running. I lay very still, constantly aware of any ectopic heartbeat that would upset my rhythm, wondering if I would even wake up in the morning. It's not something I'd ever really contemplated before, but now it was in the forefront of my mind. I thought about my parents sleeping in the next room. I knew they were feeling anxious too, each time that I arose to go to the bathroom, my mother would call out to see if I was OK. I decided to be logical about it. My heart had usually been steady overnight while I was in hospital and there was no reason why it wouldn't be the same at home.

The next day, we got up and had breakfast. I stayed in my bathrobe and slippers. The shock of leaving the cocoon of the hospital had taken its toll. My heart was beating out of my chest, and I couldn't get comfortable. I had started to perspire profusely and had turned a distinct shade of ochre yellow. I tried to lie in bed, but my heart felt very unsteady. I finally got up and went into the living room to sit with my father. My mother was just leaving the flat to buy some groceries for lunch and they both looked rather worried wondering what they should do. I took my blood pressure, and the machine showed an irregular heartbeat, but I decided to keep it from my parents as I didn't want to worry them further.

After standing up and moving towards the TV, I noticed a pile of DVDs on the floor. Amongst the numerous movies that visitors had kindly brought to the hospital, I found an episode of *Everybody Loves Raymond* and inserted it into the DVD player.

'Let's watch *Raymond*,' I said to my father trying to appear normal and hoping a bit of comedy would calm everything down. It had worked in hospital, so why not here? After about an hour, my mother returned with the shopping to see us both on the sofa laughing. I took my blood pressure again and the rhythm was back to normal. At that moment, I decided that watching comedy every morning was good for my health, a sort of happy pill, and I have done it ever since. Furthermore, numerous studies have shown that laughter has the power to relieve pain, boost the immune system, ward off cardiovascular disease, and reduce stress. In fact, laughter is both a muscular exercise and a breathing technique and it's the best natural medicine there is. Of course, some people may be in the placebo group!

Professor White was now back from an overseas trip, and I had an appointment to see him the following day at his private clinic in Harley Street. I had lost a lot of muscle while in hospital and looked extremely pale and fragile. He was very reassuring, and I felt safe in his care. Polly, the phlebotomist, took my blood to make sure I could withstand the steroid treatment. She was quite a character and each week that I attended she would be sporting a different psychedelic hair colour. My next appointment was with Dahlia, the cardiac physiologist, a petite lady with dark curly hair. She performed an excellent echocardiogram and for the first time it was not painful. She then called in Professor White to review my results. I had fluid around the heart, a dilated right ventricle, fibrosis in the left ventricle and multiple ectopic beats. It appears that some people are unaware of ectopic beats; I don't know how, because for me it felt like someone playing the maracas in my chest and I could feel every single one. There was such a caring attitude and expertise amongst all the staff at this clinic which finally allowed me to exhale, relax and let them take care of me.

As I left the room, I noticed a sign with the clinic's very sensible mission statement:

MISSION STATEMENT

1. To be friendly, helpful, and welcoming
2. To introduce ourselves by name and role, and explain what we do
3. To give each person our full attention
4. To anticipate the needs of our patients and visitors
5. To take time to listen and find out what people really want and need
6. To respond promptly and do what we have promised
7. To be well-informed and pass on information
8. To treat everyone with respect, apologising if appropriate
9. To offer to help – not wait to be asked
10. To find someone to help if we aren't able to

Later that morning, my father's best friend, David, called to see how everything was going and to say he was having some tests. He had received several ECGs at the local doctor's surgery and the nurse had told him to buy bigger socks as the elastic was digging into his lower legs. I tried to encourage him to go along to the ER and have his heart checked out properly, but he didn't want to put anyone to any trouble and said he would be fine.

As the days and weeks passed and the corticosteroids began to take effect, I started to feel better, my ejection fraction increased, I began to get some colour in my cheeks and my knees were no longer blue. I felt like I had more energy and a new lease of life. I had also started to wear the 'Zoll LifeVest' and felt reassured that it would keep me safe. The staff at the clinic were incredibly kind and supportive. There is a research unit at Harvard University set up specifically to investigate the placebo response. They have found that simple things, such as using positive words, creating a reassuring environment, and crucially ensuring that a patient trusts the doctor, can all improve the response to treatment.

As I attended the clinic one morning, Polly commented that I looked much better.

'I thought you were a "gonner" when I saw you that first day,' she said chuckling. 'You were such a terrible colour!'

She was always making me laugh, whilst doing a sterling job of taking my blood, a true expert. It hadn't always been like that with other practitioners, so rough that it sometimes felt like the needle would come out of my arm on the other side. I asked her what her secret was.

'Gentleness never went out of fashion,' she replied modestly.

'I wish you could train everyone how to take blood. It would make such a difference,' I commented.

She smiled modestly. I don't think she received many compliments, but I thought she deserved it. As soon as she received the results of my blood tests, she would send them through to me. It would prove to be lifesaving!

After my appointment, I picked up a range of brochures concerning the heart that were displayed in the clinic so that we could give them to my father's friend, David, and I joined my father who was sitting in the coffee shop waiting for me. He looked somewhat out of sorts.

'Did you have a hot chocolate?' I asked, knowing something was wrong from his facial expression?

'No,' he said, 'I was waiting for you, why don't you get us both one?'

I mentioned that I had picked up the brochures for David, left them on the table and went to buy the drinks.

When I got back, it looked as though my father had been crying.

'What's wrong?' I asked, not knowing what it could possibly be.

'Sit down,' he said and then found it difficult to find the words.

'What is it?' I said, now getting more and more concerned.

'It's David,' he said, 'he's died'.

I sat there in disbelief. What a massive blow. Here was my father looking after me with a heart problem and he had just lost his best friend by a massive heart attack in his sleep.

He later recounted that a friendly nurse from the clinic had passed by, noticed that he was getting upset after hearing the news, and had stayed with him for a while to comfort him. I was so grateful that we were in such a caring environment. Kindness truly is a universal panacea.

Along with the intense sorrow, I felt such a sense of injustice. It was clear that David had been suffering from serious heart failure and that his swollen ankles were a sign of this. The only advice he had received was to go and buy bigger socks!

Later that week my father drove me to our family home and my parents went to the funeral. David's brother, Peter, had also been suffering similar symptoms and I encouraged him to go and seek help as soon as possible. He ended up having a successful quadruple bypass.

As I needed to return to London for my ongoing care, my mother and father took it in turns to stay with me at my apartment, each one occasionally returning home to look after their affairs. I went for my first walk with my father, but only managed to reach the corner before having to return home. Over the many weeks that followed, we gradually built up to reach the next corner, and then the park, and then the first bench and eventually I was able to do one lap of the park and then two and so on. As time went by, I developed a routine of having an early morning walk in the park every day and it helped to increase my strength.

During one of the weeks when my mother was staying with me, I got dressed as usual and put on my 'LifeVest.' The electrodes were very uncomfortable at times, and I felt the need to dress in such a way to conceal the apparatus from public view. As we were preparing to leave the apartment, I popped into my bedroom to retrieve my papers which were in a drawer beside my bed. As I leant forward, suddenly a loud siren sounded as though there were a fire engine in my bedroom.

'Quick, quick,' I shouted as my mother came running from the other room.

'GET THE BATTERY OFF, GET THE BATTERY OFF,' I said with panic in my voice as I struggled to disengage the 'LifeVest' before it administered an electric shock.

We sat on the bed and regained our composure. It felt like we had just defused a bomb. It turned out that I had inadvertently removed one of the arm straps when I had taken off my cardigan and the electrodes had lost contact with my heartbeat and thought I was having a cardiac arrest. It was enough to give me one!

My ejection fraction eventually improved enough for me to take off the 'LifeVest'. It took a very long time, however, before I would feel comfortable walking in the street surrounded by lots of people. I felt an intense feeling of vulnerability, almost like a fawn with a broken leg, unable to run away. On a couple of occasions, I froze as my heart was beating uncontrollably and the onslaught of pedestrians was adding to my distress. I decided to change my route and would go out of my way to walk on quieter streets where I knew I would not need to negotiate, and be jostled by, other passers-by.

When my parents finally went home, Maria came to stay for a few days. I started to cook more elaborate dishes as I'd watched so many cookery programmes during my time in hospital. As I honed my culinary skills, I took great pleasure in being able to offer a tasty meal by way of thanks to my many friends who had helped me. Antonio Carluccio once said, 'to give food is to give love', and I agree with him.

My Results

Ejection Fraction: 39%,
one week after taking prednisolone
Ejection Fraction: 42%,
two weeks after taking prednisolone
Cardiac High Sensitivity Troponin T: 20 ng/L
BNP (NT-proBNP): 5150 ng/L
25-Hydroxy Vitamin D: 45nmol/L

CHAPTER 9

"You can easily judge the character of a man by the way he treats those who can do nothing for him."

Goethe

Dr. Noble had been contacting my employer's Human Resources Department (HR) on my behalf while I was in hospital and provided the statutory sick notes. However, it was now becoming clear that I would not be able to return to work with a heart function that was so impaired. One morning I received a call from Gary Bartlett, the HR manager from my office.

'Hello Kayte,' he said, 'how are you?'

As I sat there wearing my 'LifeVest', and I anticipated what he was about to say, I could feel my chest tightening and my heart rate increase. The company had now ceased paying my salary and I was becoming more concerned about my finances.

'I'm holding steady, thank you,' I said apprehensively.

'I wonder if I might come and see you to discuss how we take things forward,' he said.

We agreed that he would come to my apartment the following afternoon. I had worked with Gary for about four years and had helped him on several occasions navigate some difficult situations with Nigel. However, during this phone call it was obvious he was wearing his HR manager hat and had clearly been briefed to assess the situation.

Before he arrived, I had a brief phone call with Maria, who worked in HR at another company, and she was concerned that I would be seeing Gary on my own. I foolishly thought that the company would behave with integrity and so I declined her offer to be at the meeting with me, particularly as I didn't want to inconvenience her as she worked so far away.

Gary arrived at my apartment with cakes for afternoon tea, and this gesture, along with his desire to conclude the matter quickly as he was about to leave his current position to go and work in Dubai, lured me into a false sense of security. In this unguarded moment, I mistakenly thought that, in the circumstances, the company would behave honourably and do the right thing.

However, Nigel was not predisposed to treat me with compassion and sent Pandora to visit me next, which only made matters worse. I ended up having to hire an employment lawyer to fight my case, which turned out to be a particularly stressful endeavour.

I reached out to Frank Willard to ask his advice, but as he was no longer on the board, he could only recommend that I write to some of the other board members. However, being true to form they merely closed ranks. Nigel's lawyers fought relentlessly for many months, and I found it very distasteful as well as incredibly unkind. I was wearing a 'LifeVest' for most of that period, and I was dismayed at the extent of Nigel's obduracy. Maria felt that my health would not improve until the matter was settled.

Frank called me to ask how it was going. I had to tell him that it was now in the hands of lawyers as I was not well enough to fight the case on my own.

'This is something that should have been concluded in 20 minutes,' he said, 'Nigel's behaviour is most regrettable but sadly I am not surprised.'

Knowing Nigel as well as I did, having observed him for a considerable time, I remembered that his favourite expression was one by Winston Churchill, but he failed to understand the spirit of the quote.

'Never give in. Never give in. Never, never, never, never – in nothing, great or small, large or petty – never give in.'

However, he always missed off the ending:

'Never give in, except to convictions of honour and good sense.'

It would have been seemly to have settled my departure in a mature and compassionate manner, however, it was not to be. The impasse finally broke when Nigel discovered that his emails were still being delivered automatically to my BlackBerry. The heady scent of 'Schadenfreude' which flowed throughout his emails about me had forced his hand to bring the matter to a conclusion and capitulate.

Some time later, my good friend Rupert called me with news he thought might be of interest to me. He had moved jobs and was now working for a financial institution in the City. By sheer coincidence, it just so happened to be one of the firms that had invested in the company Nigel was running. Nigel's final hours as chief executive played out in a private meeting room of Rupert's company after Nigel was summoned to their offices for a meeting with four major investors. They presented him with a list of demands including his resignation. By way of compromise,

Nigel agreed to step down but only if he could spin it as retirement. Ironically, despite what had been printed in the newspapers, I was one of very few people to know the real story. It really is a small world!

After many months of blood tests and multiple hospital visits, I was finally allowed to take off the 'LifeVest'. Additionally, as the matter concerning my former employer had now concluded, my parents thought a trip overseas might be beneficial to my health, and as it was early December, the weather in England was cold again. We sought a destination that was not too far away, and which might offer some warmer weather. We decided to go to Paphos in Cyprus, a picturesque seaside town, steeped in history and with a long promenade beside the water. I was very swollen from the steroids and still looked incredibly unwell, but a change of scene was something to look forward to. We travelled there by plane, a four-hour journey and stayed at a family-run hotel by the sea. The Cypriots were very friendly and hospitable, and we were fortunate to have rooms with balconies so we could enjoy the pleasant weather without having to go to the pool.

I walked along the promenade every morning with my parents, taking in the sea air and delighting in the morning sunshine. There were beautiful, fragrant lemon trees along the route and the tranquil atmosphere was a welcome change of environment. I even managed to do some gentle yoga, although some of the poses had to be modified as I was not supposed to put my arms above my head for long periods of time.

One day, while I was sitting on the balcony, I received an email from Jeff, my friend in New York. He was doing much better and had taken a trip to Arizona. His email read:

Hello Darling Kayte,

Jeff here in Sedona, Arizona. Beautiful as ever.

I had the most hilarious experience in a yoga class in Phoenix this week at the hotel. It was a kundalini class, and the teacher was interested in energizing, not relaxing us. She shouted commands only one notch below the sound of a distressed subway train. Not an unscripted analogy because she insisted we all make loud chugga-chug noises to stimulate our chakras or something. I seem to remember something about awakening our energy bodies, like a runaway train. Then while we would be doing heavy forced breathing in pretzel-like positions that were neither standard Yoga postures nor therapeutic in any way, she would explain the effect of this non- posture on each and every organ of the body, always in her strident screaming voice. (If you have ever been to India and heard the music they play on city buses, this was worse.) But most distracting of all was how much of an obsessive-compulsive she was. She sat on an alpaca mat she had unrolled and rolled over and over till it was just right, each time lovingly refolding it as if it were a religious garment. She set before her a rolodex file, a stack of paper memos held by paper clips, a travel clock, a back-up clock, (very odd) a sand egg timer and a white plastic thingy-thing of unknown purposes. She would touch and move these items continuously. When she flipped the rolodex to find her next non-therapeutic, not-Yoga position, oh no!!!!!- the rolodex would move a nano-

> millimetre to the side, setting off a frenzy of moving all the other items just a bit to end with the same relative spacing and familiar positioning of the objects, all the while continuing to yell the breathing railroad cadence.
>
> Can't wait for a NY yoga class next week!
>
> On a positive note, all is well here and I'm feeling great. Weather great. Hiking is amazing in Sedona
>
> Lots of love,
>
> Jeff

I read the hilarious email and smiled, feeling so happy that my dear friend was back to his old self and his chemo treatment had been successful. It gave me hope that even in the darkest days good things can still happen.

My Results

Ejection Fraction: 42%
Cardiac High Sensitivity Troponin T: 13 ng/L
BNP (NT-proBNP): 3090 ng/L
25-Hydroxy Vitamin D: 70nmol/L

CHAPTER 10

"Synchronicity is an ever-present reality for those who have eyes to see."

Carl Jung

In the February of the following year, my parents went to visit my brother in Australia, and I decided to go back to the same hotel in Cyprus. I appeared to be holding steady and although I was still taking high-dose steroids, I felt somewhat stronger. This would be my very first trip on my own since the onset of my illness, and I felt comfortable knowing that I would be going back to a familiar place with friendly people. I hoped to do some more yoga and continue walking beside the sea every day, like I had on the first visit. The food was delicious and although I didn't add any salt to my meals, I hadn't realised that, as is the custom universally in restaurants and particularly in Cyprus, most of the dishes were made with huge quantities of salt. Consequently, after three weeks, I had become visibly bloated and my ankles were starting to swell.

On the last day of the holiday, I came back from a yoga class and entered my hotel room. I stopped suddenly in my tracks and noticed small fragments of glass were scattered over the floor in front of me. As I went further inside, I realised most of the glass was in the bathroom. The shower door had exploded all over the floor and had scattered the glass everywhere. It was now the second time that this had happened to me, firstly, in France with Virginia and now here. I stood there for a moment flabbergasted and questioned how on earth it had occurred again. Housekeeping came to clear up the debris and I ordered a very light dinner from room service as I was feeling rather bloated.

As I sat there, eating my supper, I received another email from Jeff. However, this time it was not good news. He'd had a relapse and was entering a drug trial but wasn't sure if he would get the experimental drug or the placebo. It was quite a shock and brought me to tears. The bad news combined with the earlier explosion had now rendered me very ill at ease.

The following morning, I left for the airport. As I started to walk around the departure hall, I realised that I was only able to walk very slowly. Suddenly I started to panic, believing I was going to miss my flight. I tried to hurry, but no matter how hard I tried, I had to keep stopping every few steps to get my breath back. I remember thinking that if a lion had escaped and entered the terminal, I would have been a tasty snack! After an interminable struggle to cross the concourse and reach the departure gate, I turned the corner to find a huge number of Argentinian soldiers who were taking the same flight back to London. I smiled thinking of Joaquin. I hadn't needed to rush after all and was able to take a seat, relax and get my breath back.

As I boarded the plane, I went to find my seat next to a gentleman who kindly helped me to put my bag in the overhead compartment. I had learnt to become a little less independent and to ask people if they would kindly assist me, and most of the time it worked. As we started out on the four-hour flight to London, the man introduced himself.

His name was John Nathaniel and he was currently living in Australia but travelled regularly to Cyprus, London, and New York on business. We had an interesting conversation and I told him a little about my recent heart problems.

'I think you need to have a conversation with God?' he said suddenly.

I was somewhat taken aback. Although I had gone to a religious school, I no longer went to church regularly but had always felt a spiritual presence which I couldn't really explain. He asked if I lived near a church, and I confirmed that there were many in my neighbourhood.

As the hours passed, we talked about a variety of interesting topics and the time just flew by.

'It sounds like you should seek a second opinion,' he said at one point while we were talking about my cardiologist. 'It's always good to try something new if you feel your progress has stalled.'

I mentioned that I hoped to go to the Mayo Clinic and meet Dr. Leslie Cooper, who had kindly helped me over the phone when I had been in hospital.

'I think that's the right thing to do,' he said, almost as though he had been tasked to convey these important messages to me. It's interesting how a brief conversation with a stranger may help point you in a different direction.

He asked me how I was travelling home from the airport and how I would manage my bags. Although I had booked a porter service, when we arrived at the conveyor belt at London Heathrow they were nowhere to be found. He was genuinely concerned and stayed with me, carrying my bags to the arrivals hall and when we finally caught up with the pre-booked taxi driver, I offered to give him a ride into London. He brought my bags to the front door of my apartment and then took the cab to his hotel. I was so grateful because, with hindsight, I realised I would not have managed to carry all the luggage on my own. The challenges of international travel would not have fazed me at all in the past, but now I realised that I was much more vulnerable, and he appeared to sense it. Looking back, he can only be described as my guardian angel.

I went to the bathroom and looked at myself in the mirror. I had transformed into a rather plump individual with bright red cheeks that looked as though I had been digging potatoes on a cold day in the middle of November. As I sat on the sofa in my living room, I realised my ankles were enormous. I texted Dahlia to ask her advice and she thought perhaps I had eaten too much salt. I spent all weekend purging my diet and ate lots of watercress soup (see recipe page 221) which reduced the ankle swelling considerably. On the Monday morning, Professor White was waiting to see me downstairs at the hospital and looked rather concerned. The echo examination Dahlia had just performed had shown a significant decrease in my ejection fraction and it was now only 33%. I had also developed a severe tricuspid regurgitation, which means that the right ventricle was so stretched with the excess fluid that the leaflets were no longer closing properly and the blood was flowing backwards. It appeared that a three-week, high-salt diet had caused a significant amount of damage. I was very distraught as I had not realised that such a small variation in diet could wreak such havoc on my little heart. It would be a year before I managed to improve my ejection fraction to 39% but unfortunately, to this day, it has never returned to 42%.

The following day, I called Serena to see how she and Harry were doing and to say that I was back from Cyprus.

During our conversation I mentioned that the shower door had exploded in my hotel room, and this was now the second time it had happened to me. Within five minutes of ending the call, Serena phoned again.

'Hello Kayte, I've just spoken to Harry about your exploding shower doors, and he said you must go and see Matthew Manning.'

'Who's Matthew Manning?' I asked, having never heard the name before.

'Harry interviewed him once when he was working as a journalist and had been impressed and intrigued by him,' she said.

I was fascinated and looked him up on the internet. I discovered he was a renowned healer, and one particular endorsement caught my eye. It was written by Professor Karol Sikora, an eminent oncologist:

'Matthew has a remarkable track record of working at the interface between body and soul. His knowledge is outstanding in both breadth and detail.'

I concluded that if medical professionals were endorsing him, what did I have to lose? Perhaps the exploding shower door was not merely a coincidence but a strong message that I should go and seek his help. At this point, although I was following all the medical advice and taking large amounts of medication, I was keen to find something else with fewer side effects which might help me on my journey to recovery.

I set about writing Matthew Manning an email and within a short space of time I received a reply. He said that he had helped one other person in the past with cardiomyopathy and thought he might be able to help me. I made two appointments on consecutive days and booked a hotel to stay overnight. I travelled by train and stayed in a quaint bed and breakfast. Matthew lived in a picturesque village in the South of England, and it seemed to have a friendly atmosphere.

From my research, I discovered that hands-on healing is a non-invasive practice which seeks to balance all aspects of well-being – physical, emotional, mental and spiritual. The treatment session was both relaxing and gentle, and I experienced a very powerful heat sensation around my heart as Matthew administered the healing. I found him very interesting and was impressed by his thoughtful approach. I went again a few months later and found both visits tremendously helpful. It is very difficult to measure the benefits of such treatment in conventional terms, but I strongly believe that many influences on the human body are often not fully understood in conventional medicine and treatments such as this often play an important role in one's recovery.

As the weeks went by, I kept in close contact with Jeff, my dear friend in New York, while he was on his new treatment and decided I would like to send him a nice gift. We had both enjoyed all sorts of music over the years and I decided to make the equivalent of what was formerly known as a 'mixtape', which of course is now called a playlist. I took great pleasure in gathering all my favourite tracks from my music collection, blending each track together seamlessly on my laptop and putting them in a specific order. By the end I had created a playlist that would last 10 hours. I downloaded it onto a mini-iPod and sent it to New York firmly sealed in a little red envelope, together with the download instructions.

Of course, within only a few years, making a playlist has now become much easier and may be uploaded to streaming services directly.

If any reader would care to listen to some of my favourite music, the playlist I made for Jeff may be found on Spotify. Just type 'Kayte Alexander' or 'The Unexpected Jeff's Mixtape' in the Spotify search bar to access the playlist. You may also click on the direct link within the playlist section of my website: www.kaytealexander.com.

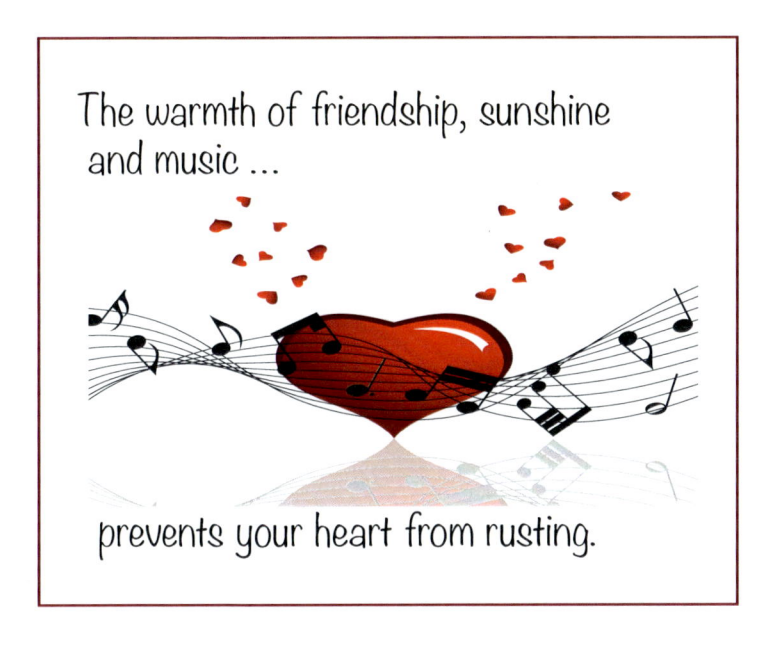

The warmth of friendship, sunshine and music ... prevents your heart from rusting.

My Results

Ejection Fraction: 33%
Cardiac High Sensitivity Troponin T: 25 ng/L
BNP (NT-proBNP): 3700 ng/L
25-Hydroxy Vitamin D: 80nmol/L

CHAPTER 11

"I've learned that people will forget what you said, people will forget what you did, but people will never forget how you made them feel."

Maya Angelou

As the months rolled by and I continued to try and improve my ejection fraction, I thought about the conversation I'd had with John Nathaniel on the airplane a few months earlier and decided to organise a trip in mid-June to the Mayo Clinic in Rochester, Minnesota, where Professor Leslie Cooper was working. My parents were now back from Australia, and they kindly agreed to go with me, as it would be such a long journey. I was hoping it might also be possible to combine the trip with another visit to see Jeff in New York. Luckily, he was now on the experimental drug, having been placed on the placebo at the beginning of the trial for a couple of months and which, obviously, had been totally ineffective. However, the new drug had shown great promise and it appeared he was finally going in the right direction. I planned to stay in New York with my parents for a couple of nights before travelling through Minneapolis to Rochester.

I emailed Jeff to finalise the arrangements and was very much looking forward to seeing him again, although I did warn him that I would look quite different. As he travelled from Connecticut to New York by train, he popped into my hotel which was located next to the station to collect me the morning after I arrived. Jeff was waiting for me as I exited the lift, sitting in the lobby on one of their futuristic chairs beside a majestic bronze statue.

'Well, you're one of the best-looking sick people I've ever seen,' he said as he smiled at me and gave me a huge hug.

Jeff always had the most amazing ability to make you feel like a million dollars, despite what life had thrown your way. I was pleased to see that he was looking much healthier than on my previous visit a year earlier. His hair had filled out again and he no longer had a yellow hue to his complexion. We ambled slowly along the sidewalk until we reached a cross street and then hailed a cab to his office. He had just concluded an exhibition of some of his artwork and asked me if I would like to choose a picture from the variety he had on display. I chose a beautiful woodcut of two people walking along a bridge in Bali. It reminded me of our enduring friendship. I took it back to the hotel, wondering how on earth I was going to get it back to London in one piece. In the end, I sent it from the hotel's mailroom to a friend in London for safekeeping while I was away. The hotel's mailroom wrapped it beautifully and it arrived without a scratch. Jeff and I agreed to meet for dinner later that evening as I was due to leave again with my parents the following morning on a flight to Minnesota. As we sat eating supper together and chatted about old times, I suddenly noticed a shift in his demeanour.

'Are you OK Jeff?' I said noticing he looked a little out of sorts.

'I've had a stressful day and had to deal with a difficult situation with one of my suppliers,' he said trying to reassure me. 'I think I'm just a bit tired.'

After dinner, he took me back to the hotel lobby and as we said goodbye we agreed to keep in close contact while I was at the Mayo Clinic. I then went to the business centre and wrote a brief email to thank him.

> Darling Jeff,
>
> When I was young and studying French, I came across a delightful quotation which made me think of you
>
> "Celui qui arrive en ami arrive trop tard et part trop tôt."
>
> There is always so much to say... I just love you with all my heart. Thank you for such a lovely, uplifting beginning and end to my day in New York.
>
> Love, Kayte xxx

The following morning, I flew with my parents to Rochester, Minnesota connecting through Minneapolis and stayed at a delightful hotel near the Mayo Clinic. As we were settling into the hotel, I received an email from Jeff.

> Hi Kayte,
>
> Thank you for your sweet email. Please let me know how the Mayo Clinic experience was perceived by you. Any answers, changes, or confirmations in diagnosis? I'm off to Italy in a couple of weeks. With love, Jeff

After a good night's sleep, we took a cab to the clinic, but as it turned out to be only two blocks away by car, we later realised that we could have accessed it directly via a climate-controlled Skyway. It all felt very state of the art and as the driver negotiated the pristine streets with his vehicle, I had the distinct impression that we were on the film set of *The Truman Show* because it was so incredibly clean, quiet, and well maintained.

I was looking forward to having the opportunity to meet and thank Professor Leslie Cooper, the cardiologist at the Mayo Clinic who had helped me so extensively over the phone while I was in hospital. The Mayo Clinic is best known for its expertise in diagnosing complex and difficult medical cases and devising the often-complex treatments that these conditions require. As we entered the clinic, there were beautiful sculptures adorning the walls, a grand piano on the central concourse and many areas to sit, read books and spend time with family members. The whole place evoked a feeling of calm, and their motto is 'The Patient Comes First'.

Professor Cooper is one of only approximately six myocarditis experts in the world, and it was invaluable to obtain his insight because he has such an in-depth understanding of the disease. He thought the inflammation was still occurring and was very concerned about my right ventricle. We also talked about what might be causing the inflammation and he considered molecular mimicry, where a foreign antigen shares sequence of structural similarities with self-antigens, i.e., cardiac myosin. In simpler terms, molecular mimicry is a case of mistaken identity where the immune system confuses the heart cells with the virus and takes aim at the wrong target. Dr. Cooper decided to make some adjustments to my medication, and I then asked him about my prognosis, as no one had wished to discuss it in the UK. His response was quite sobering but nonetheless helpful. If my heart remained in its current state 5–10% chance of death in 1 year. 50% in 5 years. I didn't tell my parents.

My Results

Ejection Fraction: 39%
Cardiac High Sensitivity Troponin T: 15 ng/L
BNP (NT-proBNP): 3250 ng/L
25-Hydroxy Vitamin D: 85nmol/L

CHAPTER 12

"If ever there is tomorrow when we're not together... there is something you must always remember. You are braver than you believe, stronger than you seem, and smarter than you think. But the most important thing is, even if we're apart... I'll always be with you."

A.A. Milne

When I returned to London at the end of June, I was emotionally and physically exhausted after a very busy ten days in the US. We had gone through Chicago on the way back and spent Saturday walking around with my parents. The city is world-famous for its plethora of unique architectural styles, but whilst the buildings were majestic, I found the atmosphere a little unfriendly in comparison to Rochester.

About a week later, I still hadn't heard back from Jeff to an email I had written telling him all about my visit to the Mayo Clinic and decided to write again. I received his reply almost immediately.

So sorry Kayte, I did get it. I've had a rough 10 days and only now am I getting to my email. The short version is that I felt awful on Thursday when we met. By Friday night I had the shakes and a high fever. Sunday night I was admitted to the hospital with pneumonia. Terrible! Disappointing! Stayed for a week with IV antibiotic. Did not work. Left for Italy on Friday. On the beach now.

As far as your news is concerned, stay positive. I am sure they will figure out something in the next 5 years.

Love, Jeff

Oh Jeff. I'm so sorry to hear you've had a rough time. Are you feeling any better? Let me know if you need help with anything while in Italy.

I just worry when I don't hear from you as you're such a good communicator. I've just had lunch with Maria, and I showed her the lovely picture you gave me. We decided on a place to hang it so I will send you a photo when it's in situ.

Anyway, I'm glad I went to the Mayo. Professor Cooper is excellent, and they have assigned a heart failure nurse to me which is something I don't have here and it's good to have someone to help if I have routine problems.

> *I hope Italy makes you feel better. Don't hesitate to reach out if you need my help.*
>
> *Love, Kayte xxx*

Jeff sent me a few pictures from Rome and Florence and seemed to be holding steady again. We exchanged a few more emails throughout the month, and then on the very last day of July I went for my usual early morning walk in the park. I was listening to the track 'Afternoon' by Pat Metheny on my smartphone and the atmosphere in the gardens that morning was particularly memorable. There was a fine dewy mist across the vegetation as though the sun was imparting diamond dust across the landscape, and everything was sparkling.

As I strolled along in the early morning sunshine, my mind wandered off to thinking about Jeff in New York and how he was fairing. I hadn't heard from him now for about a week and so I sat on the park bench to write him an email, knowing he would see it as soon as he woke up.

> *Hi Jeff,*
>
> *Just thinking about you and wondering how you are?*
>
> *Love, Kayte xxx*

I didn't get a reply that afternoon, but the following day I saw Jeff's number and picture light up on my smartphone and rushed to answer, excited at the prospect of speaking to him again. However, instead of his familiar voice, it was someone from his office who was calling to inform me that Jeff had sadly passed away, earlier that day. They talked about sending out details for the funeral arrangements by email, but all the extra words disappeared into a fog of tears that suddenly enveloped me. As the call ended, I sat there completely stunned, unable to comprehend what I had just heard. The pain in my heart was so severe, I feared I might not survive it.

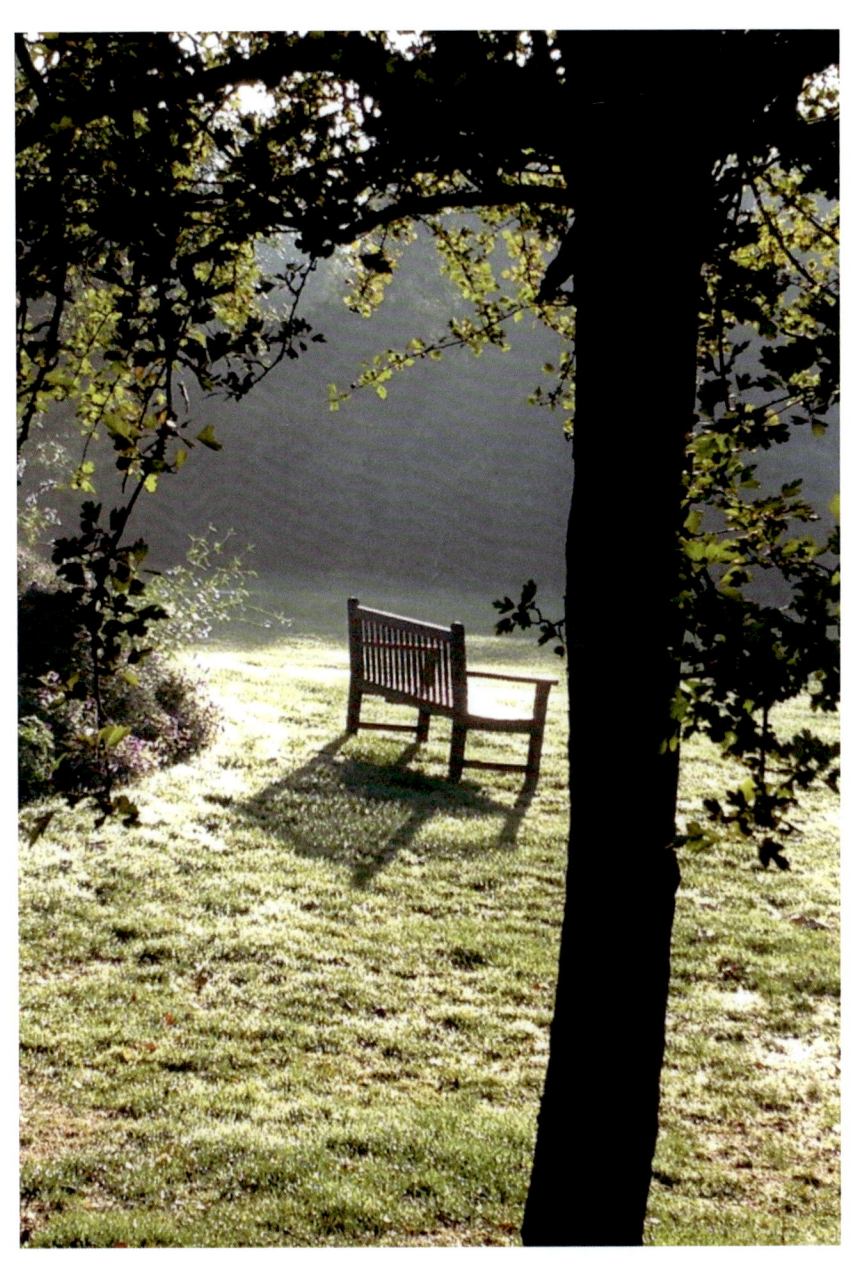

"Quos amor verus tenuit, tenebit" - Seneca

CHAPTER 14

"We can't help everyone, but everyone can help someone."

Ronald Reagan

In the spring of the following year Joaquin arrived again in London for the polo season. He and his wife were now staying in Chelsea, and although I had spoken to Joaquin on the phone many times, it would be a couple of months before I would see him in person.

Then one evening out of the blue Joaquin rang my doorbell.

'Qué pasa Dino?' he said as I answered the intercom.

'Hi Joaquin! Come on up,' I said enthusiastically.

As I opened the door and he entered the apartment planting a kiss on both cheeks, I noticed he looked rather subdued.

'I'm just watching the tennis,' I said, hoping he would be happy to watch the Federer vs Murray semi-final with me on TV.

'*Berry* well,' he said as he plopped onto the sofa.

They were playing at Wimbledon and Federer was serving beautifully. Fortunately, I had started to enjoy watching tennis again compared to the previous year when it had been impossible. At that time, my heart had not been able to withstand all the excitement but happily I had made enough progress to be able to watch it again.

As we sat there enthralled by the match, Joaquin, relaxed a little. I noticed he kept looking at his smartphone, although this was not unusual. However, I also detected a slight tension in his demeanour, and he was not his usual self. As the evening progressed, I started to feel quite ravenous.

'Are you hungry?' I asked. It was now 8pm.

'No thank you Dino. I'm waiting for Mariella. We're going out for dinner,' he replied.

'If you don't mind, I'm going to make myself an omelette as I'm starving.' He smiled and I went into the kitchen to prepare supper. As I ate the omelette, we continued to watch the tennis. Federer was playing masterfully and had already taken the first two sets 7–5, 7–5 and was up 5–4 in the third. Murray was now serving, and Federer came up with the most sublime flick of the wrist to produce a backhand winner pass to take a 0–30 lead.

'Are you sure you don't want something to eat,' I said looking for an excuse to distract myself and protect my excitable heart.

'OK,' he said.

'Are you happy with a cheese omelette?'

'I was joking Dino! Don't you want to watch the match?'

'Actually, I'm looking for an excuse not to watch it as I'm finding it too exciting,' I said.

'OK then, a cheese omelette would be nice.'

I popped into the kitchen and began rustling up a tasty supper. As the match continued, a perfect ace by Murray made it 15–30, and a killer crosscourt backhand levelled the game to 30–30. It was 9pm and the light was fading fast. Federer made a backhand service return, but it was too hot for Murray to handle, and it went to 30–40 – match point.

'Quick Dino, it's match point,' Joaquin called out.

Just as I hurried back into the room, I managed to see Federer win match point as Murray put his forehand wide. Roger Federer had played an incredible match and won in three sets 7–5, 7–5, 6–4. I was deliriously happy as Roger is my favourite player and we had both just seen one of the best matches in history. I put on my white baseball cap with RF emblazoned on the front and sat at the table grinning contentedly at Joaquin while he devoured his omelette. We chatted a little more and then he kissed me goodbye and left. I couldn't help wondering what was happening. I didn't question him about Mariella, but I had the feeling that something was seriously wrong.

About a week later, Joaquin called me again.

'Dino, are you free for lunch?' he asked.

'Sure,' I said cheerily.

'Let's go to the Italian restaurant in Holland Park.' I quickly changed my clothes and he collected me in the car.

As we sat at the table in the restaurant, Joaquin was now ready to tell me what was going on. Mariella was spending a lot of time in Italy and had basically abandoned him. They hardly saw each other any more and when she was in London, she was always working late and appeared to have disengaged. I felt genuinely sorry for him. I knew it had been a significant step to get married in the first place and within the space of only 18 months it no longer seemed to be working. We talked about what he might do, but it was clear that Mariella's mind was made up. I wondered if she had met someone else but didn't mention it as I was keen to spare his feelings. I know only too well that when one has been badly hurt, it's almost easier not to engage again. After lunch, Joaquin dropped me off at home and drove off looking rather pensive.

Later that week I hailed a cab to go to the movies.

I climbed in and sat on the racing green leather seats of the London black cab and started chatting with the driver as we sped off to Kensington High Street. As the journey progressed, I suddenly noticed a package firmly pressed against the back of the seat. I hadn't noticed it when I climbed in because the paper bag was camouflaged by the seat of the same colour. I pulled the bag towards me noticing that it had two black rope handles and was unsealed. I furtively peeked inside. There in enormous gold letters was ROLEX imprinted on a tan-coloured leather box. I slid my hand into the bag to recover the receipt. It had the name and address of the purchaser handwritten in blue ink. The script had a strong Cyrillic influence rendering it quite difficult to read, although I did manage to decipher the end of the address as 'St. Petersburg'.

I briefly toyed with the idea of giving it to the driver but wasn't confident it would get back to the owner in a timely fashion, so I decided to try and investigate myself. If I were unsuccessful, I would return it the following day to the store in Knightsbridge where it had been purchased. It then crossed my mind that perhaps the owner had simply put on the watch and discarded the packaging in the back of the cab. I waited until I reached the movie theatre and popped into the ladies' room to investigate. If there had been a fantastically expensive watch inside, I didn't want to get mugged in the process. As I opened the box, there reflecting back at me was an enormous gold Rolex with a beautiful turquoise blue face.

Oh dear, I thought. *The owner must be completely beside himself at having mislaid such an expensive item*, and I could only imagine his turmoil.

I carefully closed the package and held on to the bag for dear life. As I took my seat in the movie theatre, I tried to decipher the name on the invoice. The handwriting was proving almost impossible to read. The lights dimmed and the movie started, thwarting my first attempts at finding the rightful owner. I kept the bag firmly on my knees throughout the film, totally distracted by the investigation I was about to conduct. After watching the movie, I exited the theatre and noticed that it had started to get dark as I hailed a cab. I felt incredibly eager to get home as soon as possible so that I could start surfing the internet and find the mystery man from St. Petersburg. As I entered the apartment, I switched on the computer and spent the next hour searching for any clues the invoice might provide. Eventually, I came across a LinkedIn entry with the same name, but the text was in Russian. I managed to find the name of a company in English within the text and searched directly on their website. Finally, I came across the name again and there was an email address. I felt so excited.

Could this be the right person? And what should I say?

I decided to be a little cryptic in case it turned out to be a red herring.

> 'Sir, I got into a taxi this evening and found something on the seat which I believe belongs to you. Would you confirm that I have the right person and email me back with your telephone number so that it may be safely returned to you?'

I reread the email and pressed send.

Within minutes I received an email back with a perfect description of the package, its contents and two telephone numbers, one in Russia and one in London. It looked like all the research had paid off. I called the local number and spoke to a lady. As luck would have it, he and his wife lived just around the corner in Holland Park and agreed to come and retrieve the package.

As I went downstairs to the front door, I could see a youthful man pacing up and down. The relief on his face was a joy to behold as I handed him the package.

I felt so pleased that the search had been successful. So many people have been unexpectedly kind to me on this journey and I was glad to be able to do a little something in return.

Throughout the summer months, I started to spend a bit more time with Joaquin when he wasn't playing polo as he and Mariella were now separated, which was rather sad. He kept asking me when I was going to visit him in Argentina, and we made tentative plans for the following February. I mentioned that I was in the midst of writing a book about my illness, although Joaquin was a bit sceptical.

'Don't you think it's a bit niche as a topic? I'm not sure many people would be interested in reading it,' he said.

'Well, it's not going to be just about myocarditis, but heart failure and cardiomyopathy as well, and many millions of people suffer with that all over the world. Anyway, if Marie Kondo can write a book about tidying and sell 3 million copies, I think I can write a book about the heart,' I replied firmly.

Joaquin beamed at me, gave me a hug, and said he would look forward to reading it.

A few weeks later, we arranged a dinner at Scott's in Mayfair as a belated birthday treat. He had just returned from a trip to Madrid visiting his cousin and we met directly at the restaurant. I had bought a couple of pairs of elegant socks from the 'Paul Smith' shop in Notting Hill as a present for him, since he often looked 'sock-challenged', sporting multiple holes when he made himself at home on my sofa. As we sat at the table in the restaurant, I gave him the elegant gift box. Opening it, he smiled and asked,

'Dino, why do you keep buying me presents?'

'Because I love you,' I said, the words spilling out before I had a chance to analyse them.

'I love you too,' he said unexpectedly in return.

I sat there for a moment and smirked at him.

'Wow,' I said, 'you've never said that before! You must really mean it. You haven't even had a drink yet.'

During that summer, Joaquin was behaving a little differently and had even learned how to fly a gyrocopter. One day he decided to embark on his first cross-Channel solo gyrocopter flight. Before he left, he said goodbye, kissed me and gave me a huge hug, in case he didn't come back.

'You'd better come back,' I said, starting to feel apprehensive about this endeavour.

I am the complete opposite and more risk-averse. Adrenaline-rush adventures seem to happen to me irrespective of my desire for a quiet life. Fortunately, Joaquin made it back across the Channel safely, and a few days later I offered to make him lunch before his return to Argentina. I had wanted to cook him something special and decided to make a different recipe, salmon risotto, which I had found in a new cookery book. Unfortunately, I wasn't concentrating properly and ended up using far too much liquid. The whole dish ended up looking like wet papier-mâché. It still tasted OK, or so I thought, but when I presented it to Joaquin, somewhat disguised in a colourful bowl, he pulled a face and started playing around with it using his fork. Without any hesitation, I promptly burst into tears, surprising even myself. Joaquin just stared at me in amazement and said,

'Don't be such a baby Dino, no hay problema.'

'But it's your last meal!' I wailed, the tears streaming down my cheeks.

'I'm not Jesus Christ you know,' and we both burst out laughing.

I have never quite been able to live down that story as Joaquin often takes great delight in telling everyone in excruciating detail about my disastrous risotto. However, as he keeps coming back to enjoy my food, I don't take it too seriously, although I must say I've never dared make it again…yet!

My Results

Ejection Fraction: 39%
Cardiac High Sensitivity Troponin T: 18 ng/L
BNP (NT-proBNP): 2750 ng/L
25-Hydroxy Vitamin D: 90nmol/L

CHAPTER 15

"Life is under no obligation to give us what we expect. The unexpected makes us grow."
Irrfan Khan

In January of the following year, I caught an upper respiratory infection and developed a high fever, something that is quite unusual for me. I was prescribed an antibiotic and recovered in a couple of weeks. I had stopped the steroid in November of the previous year and appeared to be holding steady.

Joaquin was looking forward to my trip to Argentina in February. He had just started going out with someone new in his hometown, his divorce having recently been finalised. I started to prepare for my trip, buying a few items of clothing for the warmer weather and a new swimsuit. Multiple boxes of 'Octonauts' toys started to pile up in my apartment as Joaquin kept having them delivered so that I would bring them with me. I even had to buy an extra-large suitcase to carry them all.

On Friday morning, I went to see Polly at the hospital for my regular blood tests and then went home for a spot of lunch. Later that afternoon, I popped into a shop on the high street to buy a hat and received a call from Polly.

'I think something's seriously wrong,' she said. 'One of your results is extremely high.'

Knowing that the laboratory had just changed the way it now measured certain tests, I asked her which one.

'It's the troponin T,' she said, 'it's 245 ng/L.'

The highest level of troponin T I'd experienced in hospital was 131 ng/L and that was after the trauma of the heart biopsy, so 245 ng/L was off the scale and indicated a massive amount of inflammation in the heart muscle. I asked if the shop had a fax machine and Polly kindly faxed the paperwork through to me.

I looked at the results and couldn't believe what I was reading. There in black and white was a troponin T level of 245 ng/L and the normal range was supposed to be between 0–14 ng/L.

I thanked the shop assistant and left the store, jumped into a cab and went home quickly. As it was late on Friday afternoon, I didn't have any way of contacting my new cardiologist. Professor White had now changed jobs and had gone to practise in the Middle East, and I didn't want to go to the emergency room and get caught up in the hospital system all over again with people that didn't understand my history.

While I was sitting on my sofa, not quite believing that this was happening to me again, I remembered that I still had Professor Cooper's mobile telephone number. I rang it and he answered immediately.

'Hello, Dr. Cooper, it's Kayte Alexander from London. Am I disturbing you?' I asked.

'Not at all, I'm currently driving from Rochester to Jacksonville, Florida, where I will be taking up a new post,' he said in a friendly manner.

'It's not good news, I'm afraid. I appear to be in the

midst of a serious relapse. My troponin has increased to 245 ng/L.'

Once again, Professor Cooper was incredibly helpful and friendly, and I felt so grateful and fortunate that this dear man was able to help me at such a distance in my hour of need. He recommended that I repeat the blood test on Monday and see my cardiologist as a matter of urgency.

Of course, the only treatment available to me was to go back on high-dose steroids with all the accompanying side effects. Over the last three months, I had started to enjoy getting closer to my former self and losing much of the weight I had gained, but now I would be facing yet another rollercoaster of doctors' visits, blood tests, MRIs, a massive moon face and further weight gain. Although the troponin T started to reduce as soon as I commenced the steroids, for a variety of reasons there had been a week's delay in commencing the medication and, unfortunately, in this very short space of time I had become severely breathless and felt like I was back at square one again.

Furthermore, considering the severe relapse, it was highly unlikely I would still be able to go on my long-awaited trip to Argentina, despite Joaquin holding out until the very last minute to cancel. It would have been just too dangerous to embark on such a long journey on my own and I would not have felt comfortable. Eventually we both had to accept that I would not be able to travel, and I gave the huge suitcase of toys to a friend who was going to Argentina a few weeks later.

Despite the disappointment, Joaquin came back to London again for the polo season a few months later and I continued to make good progress throughout the summer. The next warm weather season in Argentina would be October and I hoped to be back on track by then.

Miraculous Magnesium...

After this very disappointing relapse, I realised that I would not be able to rely on just taking the prescribed medication to keep me well and that I needed to work harder at finding other ways to improve my health (see Chapters 20–24 for further details). As I was still experiencing multiple ectopic heartbeats otherwise known as premature ventricular contractions (PVCs), I was particularly keen to find other ways that might improve my heart failure and try to arrest the inflammation in my heart which was continually smouldering. I had spoken to multiple medical practitioners about my incessant PVCs, but they had no suggestions, and as I was unable to take beta blockers, I was told I would just have to get used to them. However, being determined to see if I could find something that might help stop the constant interruptions in my chest, I scoured the internet for any clues. I came across a few blogs which mentioned the supplement 'magnesium'. One chap, who had a normal heart function, had been plagued with PVCs and he said they were ruining his life. He had been on multiple hospital visits, but they couldn't find anything wrong with his heart. In the end, he had tried magnesium and the PVCs had miraculously disappeared. About a year later he became lazy in taking the supplement and they returned with a vengeance. After another round of hospital checks which proved inconclusive, he started the magnesium again and happily they disappeared.

As I continued to take so much prescribed medication, I needed to check that a supplement of magnesium would not be contraindicated. I was already eating foods that should have been quite high in magnesium, but many of the soils are now depleted and it is not always guaranteed that our foods will contain enough. Moreover, heart failure, steroids, stress, strenuous exercise, and the use of diuretics all deplete the body of magnesium, so it would be no surprise if I were deficient. I researched extensively and discovered that many papers had been published on the benefits of magnesium and its effect on curbing PVCs. Furthermore, Dr. Sanjay Gupta has made an excellent video about the multiple benefits of magnesium (yorkcardiology.co.uk).

I checked with my cardiologist and although the magnesium level in my blood had been at the lower end of normal, she was happy for me to give it a try. I purchased an easily assimilated liquid formulation of the mineral supplement, as magnesium gluconate, and took it every day at breakfast. Within a week, my PVCs had reduced significantly. The difference was like night and day. As the weeks went by, instead of feeling the familiar fluttering in my chest, my heart felt much happier, and I became less aware of any errant rumblings. Some might ask if it's the placebo effect, but I have forgotten to take the supplement on occasion and the PVCs have crept back unexpectedly. There have also been times when I have not been able to sleep because of the PVCs and a dose of magnesium at bedtime will invariably quieten everything down. I have also known people use it to help with atrial fibrillation and palpitations. It appears to be a very important mineral for many functions in the body as well as the heart. In general, I'm not sure that all in the medical profession appreciate the importance of magnesium. Despite being plagued by continuous PVCs throughout my illness, no one had ever recommended I take it, but from the very moment I started taking magnesium, it has changed my life.

I finally met an ER doctor whom I had to consult as an emergency a couple of years ago, and she had asked me what medications I was taking. I gave her the very long list and then said,

'Oh, and I also take 250mg of magnesium daily.'

'It's wonderful, isn't it?' she replied.

I looked at her in amazement. This was the first time that anyone had confirmed how fantastic it was.

'We use it in the emergency room setting. If anyone comes in with a funny rhythm problem, we give them magnesium and it often settles it right down.'

So, there you are, many anecdotes, and I can happily say, from my own first-hand experience, that I believe magnesium to be truly MIRACULOUS! (But always check with your doctor before taking it.)

My Results

Ejection Fraction: 37%
Cardiac High Sensitivity Troponin T: 245 ng/L
BNP (NT-proBNP): 4250 ng/L
25-Hydroxy Vitamin D: 95nmol/L

CHAPTER 16

"All journeys have secret destinations of which the traveller is unaware."

Martin Buber

After months of gradually reducing the steroids to a much lower dose, I forged ahead with booking my trip to Argentina and had a final blood test the day before I was due to leave. The results were stable and I was given the green light to travel. It would be my first solo long-haul flight since my illness, a journey of some 13 hours, and luckily, I managed to use airmiles to travel in business class so that I could keep my legs elevated.

After an uneventful flight, I arrived at the airport in Buenos Aires. Having found someone to help me put all my luggage on a trolley from the conveyor belt, I then had to attempt to take my suitcases off again to get them through an X-ray machine, one by one, while the person at border control just stood there watching me struggling. Sometimes, it's hard for people to appreciate what is going on inside the body when, from the outside you look perfectly strong and healthy, but on the inside your heart is severely damaged.

As I finally came through the exit doors into the arrivals hall, Joaquin was there waiting for me, drinking his morning macchiato. We then went to collect his car, a gigantic American vehicle with enormous wheels and loaded the luggage into the back. He planned to take me to the *Avenida 9 de Julio* so that I could see the sights and enjoy the fascinating array of architecture. Buenos Aires does not have a dominant architectural style but rather an arbitrary mixture of cosmopolitan designs, including art deco, art nouveau, neoclassical, neo-gothic renaissance, and French-Bourbon. For someone who greatly appreciates architecture, I was in for a treat. We would then have lunch in one of Joaquin's favourite restaurants before going to the farm, known in Spanish as *el campo*.

However, as we left the airport, within only a few moments we got caught up in a massive traffic jam. Motorbikes were trying to weave in and out and we stayed there for at least two hours unable to move. Joaquin was very disappointed as obviously it was not the first impression of Argentina that he had intended. However, eventually the cars started to move, and we gathered speed along the motorway. Suddenly Joaquin noticed on the digital display of his dashboard that the air pressure in both front tyres was starting to go down and as we were travelling along it was getting lower and lower. Not being aware of the types of antics which criminals use in this part of the world, I was oblivious as to why this should cause Joaquin so much concern. However, I could see by his face and flaring nostrils that something was seriously amiss as he increased his speed to try and get off the motorway at the next exit.

Fortunately, as Joaquin left the highway, we saw a 'Firestone' sign at the end of the ramp and so we were able to drive straight into the nearby garage. They hoisted the car up and discovered two screws had been inserted strategically in exactly the same position in both front tyres. Someone had obviously planned to rob us as soon as we broke down, and it's likely they had carried out the sabotage while we were sitting ducks in the traffic jam.

'You're already causing trouble,' Joaquin said as he got his sense of humour back while we waited for both tyres to be repaired.

After leaving the workshop, we made our way to the restaurant passing an imposing silhouette of Eva Perón on the Ministry of Health building. By the time we sat at the table for lunch, we were both ravenous, and Joaquin ordered two enormous steaks, which melted like butter in the mouth. We sat there chatting for a while, both grateful for having survived such a hair-raising incident. Sadly, after all the shenanigans since leaving the airport, Joaquin had no time left to show me Buenos Aires, and consequently we had to travel to the farm as soon as we left the restaurant.

Although the tyres had been repaired, the wheels on the vehicle were now severely out of alignment and any unevenness on the road surfaces transferred throughout the vehicle shaking my little heart constantly. It was deeply uncomfortable throughout the three-hour journey, and I had to keep asking Joaquin to slow down, which didn't really accord with his personality. Despite the bumps, what struck me the most about the landscape was the extreme flatness of the surrounding Pampas and the vastness of the sky.

As we finally arrived at *el campo* after the excruciatingly long and arduous journey Joaquin had all but lost his sense of humour with me. We quickly freshened up and went to meet a couple of his friends, Lauren and Chris, for dinner. Fortunately, by the time we had eaten a fantastic piece of the most delicious Argentinian beef and drunk a glass of full-bodied Malbec wine, all was forgotten and instead we were able to transform the experience into the tale of the exciting commencement to my vacation.

The next day, I awoke to birds singing and the sun piercing through the curtains in my bedroom. Joaquin's girlfriend, Valentina, had arrived to take me to the supermarket so we could find some supplies for breakfast. She was pretty, blonde, and petite with a kindly disposition and had known Joaquin since childhood. They had been in the same class at school together and while she had been quite studious, Joaquin had apparently spent most of his time sitting at the very back of the class being naughty which, I must say, did not surprise me at all.

Joaquin has a very big family and had arranged for an *asado* for later that day. *Asado* literally means barbecue, but the translation doesn't do it justice as it is, in fact, often a much more elaborate event and social gathering with copious amounts of delicious cooked meats, invariably turned on a spit and served with accompanying salads, lots of red wine and the famous chimichurri sauce (see recipe page 233). Many of his cousins, aunts and uncles had arrived and were preparing for the family meal on the largest table I have ever seen. I met Joaquin's parents who were delightful and learned that his mother had been an English teacher. She spoke the most beautiful English with hardly an accent. I also met his grandmother who was 100 years old, and Joaquin took great delight in introducing me to her as 'one *dinosaurio* to another'.

We all thoroughly enjoyed the *asado* and while eating a particularly decadent dessert Chris called out to Joaquin, 'How do you say naughty in Spanish?'

'I don't think he understands the meaning of the word,' I immediately quipped, and we all burst out laughing.

They were a very warm, friendly group of people and made me feel at home instantly. I also had the chance to meet and thank Dr. Love, the cardiologist who had helped me while I was in hospital as well as Dr. House, Joaquin's internist cousin. Later that afternoon Joaquin's mother asked if I would like to go with them to their local Catholic church as the Father, a famous healer, would be giving a special Sunday evening service and they were confident that he would be able to help with my heart. I jumped at the chance, and his mother, aunt and uncle whisked me into their car and off we sped into town. Joaquin would come to collect me later.

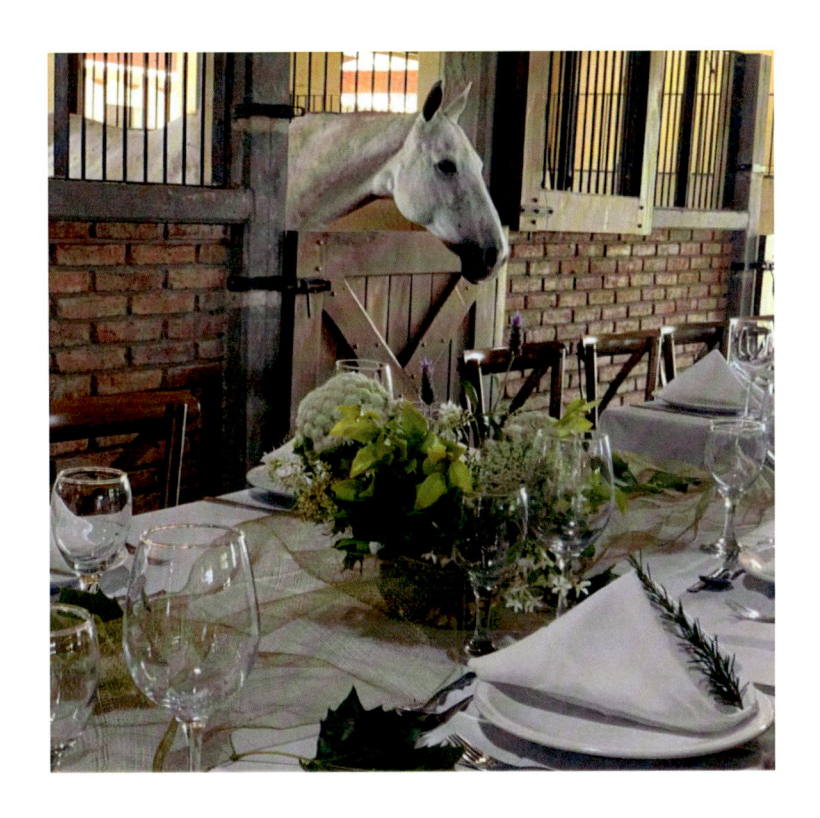

As I stood there listening to the sermon in Spanish, I looked around at all the people who were lining up, hoping to receive a healing blessing from Father Ignacio. I could see him from a distance, and he appeared to have a very kind face and gentle demeanour. After the sermon, we were divided into groups, and I went down to the front and awaited my turn. The priest had so many people to see that night and it took such a long time that it was around midnight before I was able to meet him. I stood opposite Father Ignacio, and he spoke to me in perfect English, having spent some of his earlier years preaching in North London. We spoke about my heart and chatted for a long while. I found his insight extremely moving, and tears flowed as I listened to his kind words. Although many people were around us, it felt as though we were both alone in talking with God. After the healing, he gave me a special holy *medallita*, suggested that I drink the holy water while staying in Argentina and walk on the grass barefoot every day. (See note page 255.)

As I joined Joaquin's family again in the church, they marvelled at how long Father Ignacio had spent with me. He usually had a very short amount of time with each person, but in my case, it had lasted much longer than usual, and I was so grateful to have had the opportunity to experience such a truly special moment with him.

A few days later, Joaquin went to collect a little puppy. He was a handsome Weimaraner and had the most amazing pale celadon green eyes, a short, sleek silver-grey coat, gigantic floppy ears, and enormous paws. Joaquin had decided to call him Floki, and the young puppy had travelled back to the farm in Joaquin's massive vehicle, hardly batting an eyelid throughout the journey. He seemed to have a good nature and was already house-trained. Joaquin prepared a bed for him to sleep in the barn and during the day he would relax in a plush cushion outside on the veranda, while benefitting from the shelter of the overlying roof. At first, he would cry at night and did not want to be left on his own, and very occasionally I would bring him into my room to comfort him, but Joaquin did not want me to spoil him as he was a farm dog.

As he liked lots of exercise, I started to take him on longer and longer walks. Gentle walking was good for my heart and Floki enjoyed the individual attention. It was also a clever way to distract him from digging holes everywhere. When the polo field was empty, I would try to go for a long walk, building up the distance every day and finally managed to walk from one end of the field to the other, throwing a soft rubber ball for Floki to fetch to keep him interested and get maximum exercise. I took great pleasure in teaching him how to 'sit', 'stay' and 'come', in my typical Anglo-Saxon way. He did appear to enjoy the training, and I noticed that spending time with him was beneficial to me also. Whilst on the beautifully manicured polo field I would often kick off my shoes to walk barefoot on the grass as Father Ignacio had suggested. Occasionally, Floki would get caught up with another dog on the farm and, although he was bigger than the older dog, he managed to escape rather the worse for wear, looking sorry for himself. Sadly, now he even has a few battle scars on his face to show for it.

Eventually, he acclimatised to staying in his own bed overnight but was always happy to see me in the morning when I awoke, eager for another walk. Sometimes the housekeeper would come out of her house shouting and waving her arms as Floki would love to steal any shoes he could find and place them as a prize in front of my door. It was comical trying to communicate with her, as I spoke very little Spanish, and although I tried to use a translation app, I couldn't always get a Wi-Fi signal and ended up having to use hand gestures. In the past, I'd been somewhat apprehensive of dogs after an unfortunate incident as a child when my mother and I had to climb out of a bathroom

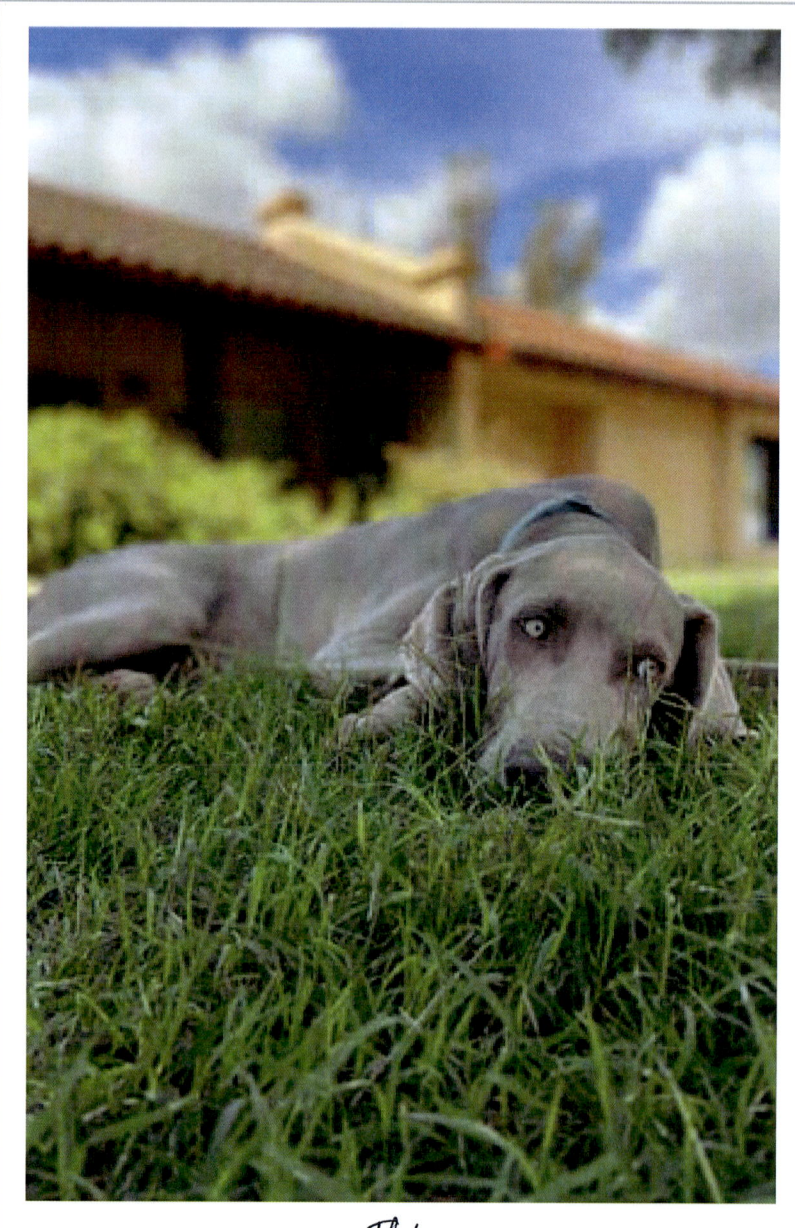

Floki

window to escape some fighting Alsatians. However, Floki's temperament was playful, and he seemed to have an innate desire to take care of me.

One day while walking around *el campo*, we came upon a gaucho (a cowboy from the South American Pampas) who was just bringing a young stallion into the centre of a round pen. I wondered if he was going to attempt 'Join-Up', a technique developed by Monty Roberts many years ago, which I had seen on TV but had never seen in person. Floki was now exhausted after his run, and I was able to sit watching for a while with Floki dozing at my feet.

The gaucho encouraged the horse to run around the pen in both directions, locking his eyes onto him and causing him to take flight, by slapping a rope on his leg. His shoulders were always square to the horse, and he continued to stare directly at him. As horses are flight animals, their first reaction to a predator is to flee using speed to escape from danger, but they cannot run for ever and will eventually slow down and reassess the situation. This is known as 'advance and retreat' and is an essential form of communication between a man and a horse, a language known as 'Equus'.

The first gesture I noticed was the horse pointing his closest ear towards the gaucho. He attempted to move a little closer towards the centre of the pen slowing down his pace slightly. The horse started to lick and chew which indicated that he was beginning to trust the gaucho and finally he dropped his head down near the soil and allowed it to bounce along. As soon as he observed all four gestures, the gaucho moved his eyes away and turned his shoulders on a 45-degree angle to the body axis of the horse. I watched him stand there motionless for a brief moment and then the horse approached him with his nose reached out nudged him in the back, known as the moment of 'Join-Up'.

The gaucho rounded his body and carefully turned around, but this time with his eyes looking down between the horse's front legs. He proceeded to rub the stallion between his eyes as a reward for 'Join-Up'. Amazingly the horse started to follow the gaucho around the pen no matter where he went. He even walked in a zig-zag pattern, while all the while the horse kept close to his shoulder. It was such a pleasure to witness and very moving.

Although horses were not indigenous to Argentina, they have become an intrinsic part of its national identity and culture. There are many equestrian sports performed throughout the entire country, but the most famous and internationally well-known is polo. Argentina has dominated this sport since it was introduced by English immigrants in the 1800s and its polo team has been the uninterrupted world champion since 1949. Chris has been a polo instructor for years and patiently introduced me to a little riding on a docile horse, although it did take quite a lot of effort just to get into the saddle. However, heart failure and riding don't really mix, and I had to be satisfied with a little trot around and a few photographs which gave the impression I knew what I was doing. The real joy was watching Joaquin, Chris, Joaquin's brother Federico and Dr. Love play regularly while I was there. It certainly is an exciting and fast-moving sport.

I had developed a routine and would begin most days watching *Seinfeld* on TV while eating my breakfast and getting my essential dose of comedy. I would take Floki for his daily walk, often watch polo, go on long drives with Joaquin, Valentina, Lauren, Chris and their son Ethan in the Pampas and eat the most delicious Argentinian steaks. However, as the weather had been unseasonably cool for the time of year, after a few weeks Joaquin decided to take us all on a trip for a long weekend to a lovely hotel in Patagonia.

San Carlos de Bariloche, usually known just simply as Bariloche, is a city in the province of Rio Negro, situated in the foothills of the Andes on the southern shores of the Nahuel Huapi Lake. It is located within the Nahuel Huapi National Park, the oldest in Argentina, stretching out over 2 million acres, and is bordered by Chile on its western side. The city is known as a major tourism centre with a variety of winter sports during the colder months and outdoor pursuits in the summer.

After travelling by plane to San Carlos de Bariloche airport, we all piled into a rental car and Joaquin drove to the hotel. We stopped off briefly to take some photographs at Cerro Campanario and marvelled at the stunning 360-degree views of the surrounding lakes and park. As we continued the journey, I noticed the most glorious scenery with snow-covered mountains and Alpine-styled architecture, which had been constructed in the 1930s and 1940s.

The hotel was majestic, perched on a bluff between the Moreno and Nahuel Huapi lakes, sitting beneath the imposing Andes mountains. Everywhere I looked the scenery was captivating, and it reminded me of some of the views in the Swiss Alps but on a much larger scale. Joaquin, Valentina and Chris played golf a few times and I went for lots of walks with Lauren and Ethan, exploring the vast hotel grounds. Joaquin also organised a few day trips so we could explore the spectacular surrounding landscape. We also walked around the town of Bariloche, visiting some of the many chocolate shops which have led to its reputation as Argentina's chocolate capital. They even have a museum dedicated to this delicacy. The city was not founded until 1902 and was originally populated by colonies of Swiss, Italians and Germans who have left their imprint on the culture and architecture. Although I had eaten some of the best Argentinian beef while at the farm, it was wonderful to be able to enjoy some delicious local seafood from the nearby lakes, trout and salmon, in particular.

As I had been having such an enjoyable time in Bariloche and my friends were obliged to return to work after the weekend, I decided to extend my stay for a short while and take the opportunity to completely relax. I would then go back to *el campo* for a few more weeks before returning to London.

CHAPTER 17

"There's only one thing that can heal the heart... Only one... It's love."

Masashi Kishimoto

A few days later, after savouring a delicious lunch of grilled salmon and a medley of steamed vegetables, I decided to go down to the pool to take advantage of the warm afternoon sun. Placing my belongings in a brightly coloured beach bag, I changed into my swimsuit and wore a lacy white summer dress with a straw sun hat edged in a rose-gold ribbon. I hadn't attempted to swim since the onset of my illness because my cardiologist had advised against it. Crossing the deserted indoor pool area, I noticed a tall metal and glass door which led outside. As I pushed open the heavy door, the hinge clanged noisily. To my left was a pristine infinity pool, perched on a deck with a spectacular view of the snow-covered Tronador mountain in the distance. Although the outside air was a little fresh, the seating area on the right was surrounded by a glass wall providing shelter from the wind. I walked over to the end of the pool and slipped off one of my flip flops to test the water. It was incredibly warm and inviting. As I walked towards one of the chairs, I noticed I was not alone. One other person was lying on a sun lounger, wearing a baseball cap, and reading a book. He seemed very relaxed and looked up briefly to acknowledge me by nodding gently before returning to his reading. I made myself comfortable and laid out a plush white towel on the sun lounger before stretching out, savouring every warm ray that penetrated my skin. Lying there was incredibly comforting and blissfully luxurious. I felt a peaceful joy as my little heart was beating gently and calmly in my chest. After a spell, I glanced in his direction and noticed that my neighbour had ventured over to the pool, then dived into the water with barely a splash. His tall, athletic body was lightly tanned, and he had wavy sandy blonde hair. He started to do laps in the pool, and I was able to watch him for a little while unobserved behind my sunglasses. As I listened to my playlist, I noticed he had lifted himself up with muscular leverage at the side of the pool, and with the towel wrapped firmly around him, he started to walk in my direction.

'Hello,' he said, 'are you here on holiday?' The timbre of his voice was mellifluous, and he had a very soft South African accent.

'Yes, I'm here visiting from London,' I said, 'how about you?'

'I'm from Cape Town and on a tour of South America. I decided to stay here a little longer as it's such an amazing place. My name's Oscar Lieberman,' and he extended his hand to shake mine.

'I'm Kayte Alexander, good to meet you,' as I grasped his hand in return. He had a confident handshake, and his skin was firm and pleasant to the touch. I also noticed he had sparkly, crystal blue eyes and his eyebrows were bleached blonde and met in the middle.

'Would you mind if I joined you?' he continued, 'I'm not sure where everyone is today. I think quite a few people may have checked out because of the coronavirus.'

'Yes, please do pull up a chair,' I said and asked if he would like a refreshment.

'Let me go and find someone,' he said. 'What would you like to drink?'

'Just a San Pellegrino with a slice of lime, no ice, thank you,' I replied.

As he wandered off, I looked at my smartphone to see if I might discover any news on the coronavirus. I had left the UK in mid-January and had been somewhat sheltered from what was going on in the rest of the world. The Wi-Fi signal at the farm had been erratic and it was often difficult to achieve a connection.

As Oscar strolled back with our drinks, he placed them on the little round table between the chairs and went off to collect his belongings. As he settled on the lounger beside me and picked up his drink, I said,

'You're a long way from home?'

'Yes, I'm on a sabbatical. I sold my business and am trying to decide what to do next.' He looked youthful but might easily have been in his mid-to-late fifties.

'How about you?' he asked. He had an intensity in his expression which conveyed a captivating prejudice in one's favour. It was a little unnerving.

'I've been visiting a friend not far from Buenos Aires. He has a farm there and is a professional polo player.'

'Do you play polo?' he asked.

'No, but I do have a great picture which looks like I do,' I said laughing, as I showed him the staged photograph of me holding a polo stick on horseback which was snapped at the start of the holiday.

'Wow, that looks like fun,' he said. At this point, I was loath to mention my illness and did not wish to temper an otherwise delightful conversation.

We sat there chatting for a long while and I was surprised at how easily our conversation flowed. Although we had only just met, we had a profound and mystical connection that transcended the usual pleasantries. Suddenly he stood up to go back into the pool.

'Are you coming in for a dip?' he said playfully.

I hesitated for a while, not sure what I should do. I guess now was the moment to let him know that I wasn't as strong as I once was.

'Actually, I haven't been in the water for some time,' I said gingerly. 'I've had a few health problems and I'm being extra cautious.'

He hesitated and then said,

'You're such a gorgeous woman, so vital! I'm sure you'll be fine. The water is incredibly warm and, in any event, I'm here if you get into trouble.' He was smiling broadly as he dived into the pool again and started swimming.

I was a little taken aback. I wasn't used to receiving compliments any more. Since my illness, I had felt invisible and was amazed that this complete stranger could see beyond what I had endured to the person underneath. He appeared to be reassuringly authentic. I stood up and wrapped the white towel around me. Unfortunately, my body had been ravaged by the steroids and I was not as trim as I once was. I entered the water furtively while he was swimming in the opposite direction and slid into the most glorious, silky water. It was like entering a warm bath and I started to swim, keeping close to the edge. Suddenly I felt rejuvenated as though I was tasting the magic of life for the very first time. Swimming didn't appear to make me too breathless, and I was able to glide gently back and forth a few times.

As I climbed the pool steps to exit and grabbed my towel, I felt invigorated. This was my very first swim for two years and it allowed me to feel yet another step closer to normality. I walked back to the sun lounger and wrapped myself snugly in a towelling robe. The air had developed a sharp edge in contrast to the heat of the pool and the sun was now getting lower in the sky. As I sat down, I noticed a book sitting on the table – *Who Moved My Cheese?* by Dr. Spencer Johnson. As Oscar took his seat, I said,

'How are you enjoying the book?'

'It's surprisingly interesting,' he replied, 'I think it might be quite old as it's rather dog-eared. I found it downstairs in the hotel library. There weren't too many books in English to choose from, so I think someone must have left it behind. Have you read it?'

'Yes, I have actually,' I said, 'I read it when I was on holiday in Australia many years ago. I was between jobs at the time and not sure what to do next.'

'What did you decide?' he said breezily.

I chuckled, 'I went back to London and found a job in the City for a while, working for an investment bank in the Gherkin. Who knows if that was the right decision?'

'What are you doing now?' he asked.

'I'm writing a book, but I've been stuck on the ending.'

He looked at me and smiled. 'You're so easy to talk to. Would you care to have dinner with me tonight?'

'What a lovely idea!' I said, suddenly feeling emboldened by my swimming experience. We agreed to meet in the bar for a drink before dinner at 7pm.

When I got back to my room, Joaquin was calling the hotel phone.

'Dino,' he said, sounding relieved to have reached me. 'You've got to leave the hotel tomorrow morning. Argentina is going into lockdown because of the coronavirus. I'm coming to get you at 7.30am with a little 4-seater Piper plane. I've checked and the hotel has a runway.'

I opened the envelope which I had picked up as I entered my room. It was from the hotel management confirming that all guests would need to depart the following morning.

'Do you have room for one more passenger?' I asked, 'I've met someone here and he may need our assistance.'

'Yes, Dino. No problem!' Joaquin said, always happy to help.

I quickly showered and dressed for dinner wondering if Oscar would be joining us at the farm the following day. The strongest feelings often arise from the promise of what might happen, and I started to feel a little nervous excitement as I entered the bar. The log cabin-style venue was magnificent with enormous beams across the ceiling. An amber glow emanated from the stone fireplace as the flames enveloped the burning logs. Oscar looked very relaxed as I joined him for a glass of champagne. He was wearing navy blue gabardine trousers with a crisp aqua-coloured shirt which intensified his pale blue eyes.

'You look quite lovely,' he announced in the charming lilt of his accent as he stood up to greet me.

'Thank you!' I replied, feeling a little self-conscious.

I had decided to wear a silk dress with a delicate blue and lilac paisley design together with my favourite electric blue kitten heels. He leaned forward to kiss me on the cheek, and I inhaled the refreshing spicy vetiver scent of his cologne whilst noticing the soft skin of his freshly shaven face.

Adjacent to the bar was a majestic mountain-style restaurant with exposed cypress timbers and after a relaxing moment together in the bar drinking champagne the waiter escorted us to our table. We savoured a delicious dinner of Patagonian lamb and our conversation flowed from one subject to another. Throughout the evening, a band was playing wonderful Brazilian music.

'Would you care to dance?' he asked, as they started to play a soulful bossa nova.

'Thank you,' I said softly, and we moved to a small wooden dance floor at the edge of the restaurant. He was quite a bit taller than me and had strong, muscular shoulders. Taking me in his arms, it felt very comfortable, as though we had already known each other for a very long time. Oscar had a surprisingly good rhythm and we swayed together gently to the tempo of the music.

'I know this is perhaps a little presumptuous of me,' I said hesitantly, 'but, as you know we are all obliged to leave the hotel tomorrow. Joaquin is coming to collect me by plane at 7.30am, and I was just wondering if you would like to join us?'

'That's kind of you,' he said. 'To be honest I wasn't sure what I was going to do.'

'He has accommodation where you could stay and maybe you'd like to learn how to play polo?' I added, smiling.

His blue eyes twinkled as he replied mischievously, 'I think Sniff and Scurry would approve of that idea, don't you?' He had obviously now finished reading the *Who Moved My Cheese* book.

The following morning as we stepped outside, the sun had a magnificent hazy glow, emerging softly through the dawn and announcing the promise of a beautiful day. Joaquin smiled proudly as we took our seats in the back of the aircraft and then he roared the Piper plane along the grass runway at great speed. As it carried us into the radiant sky, I felt excited at the prospect of yet another adventure and how wonderful it was TO BE ALIVE.

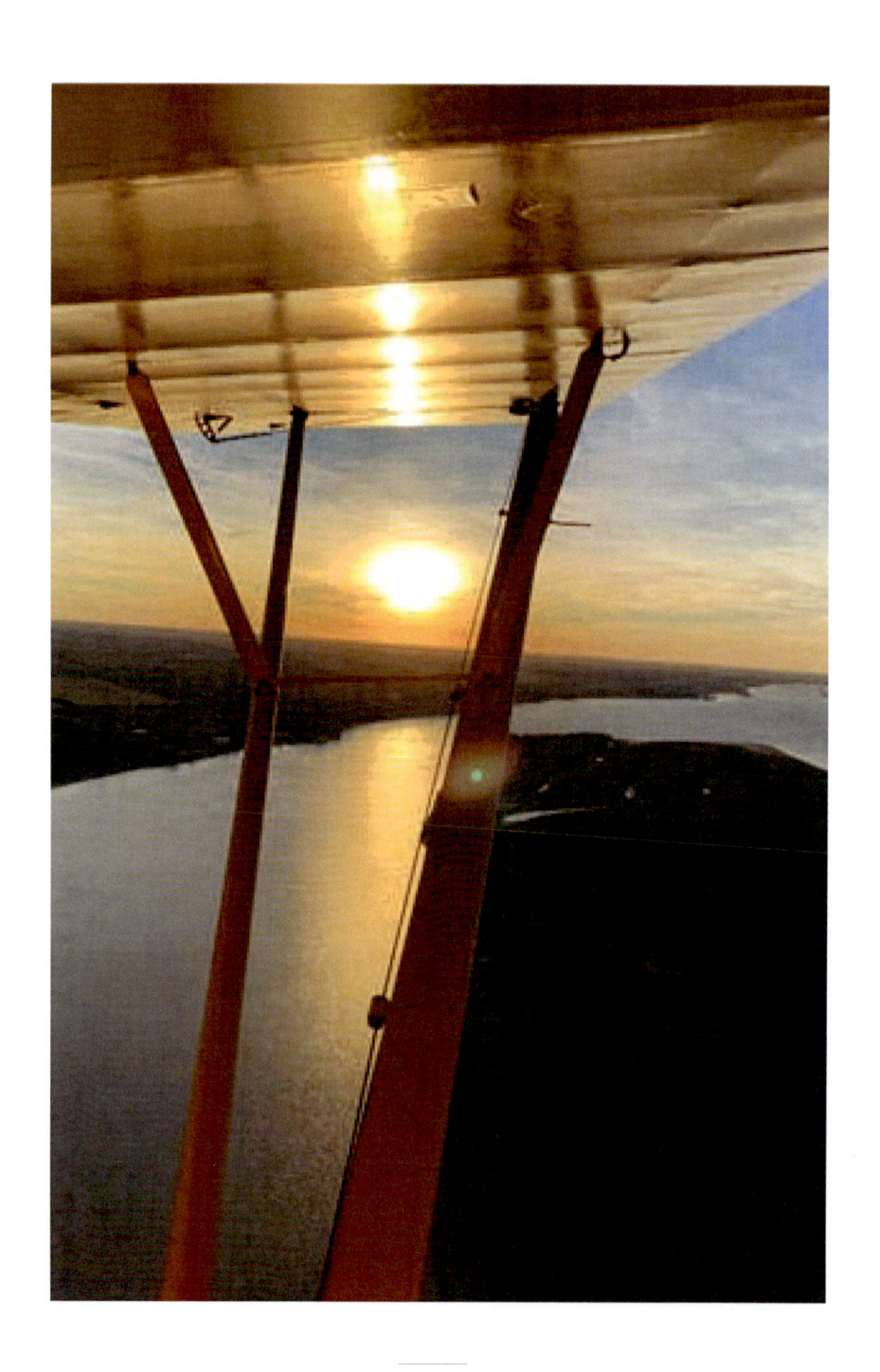

Epilogue

"If you keep a green bough in your heart, the singing bird will come."

Chinese proverb

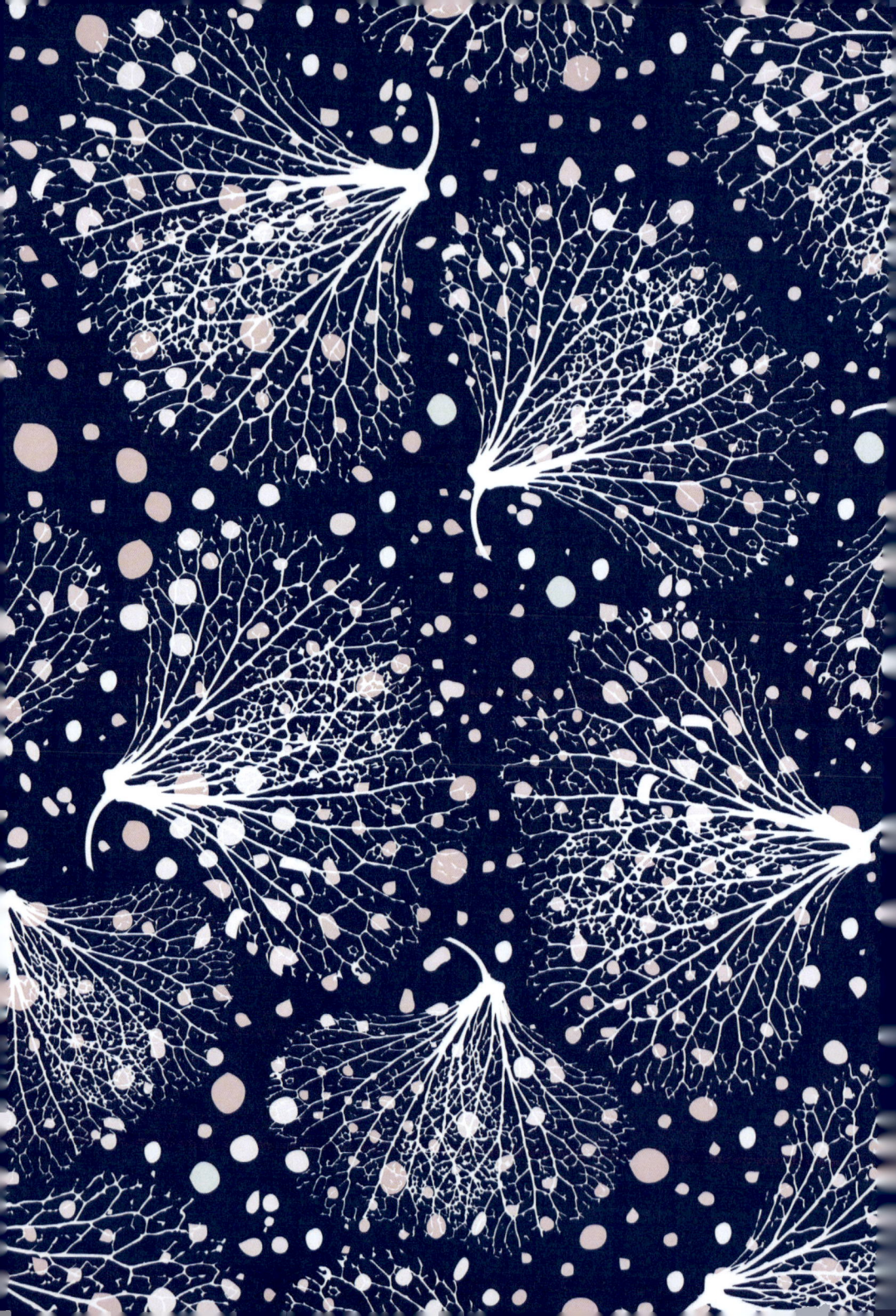

Part Two

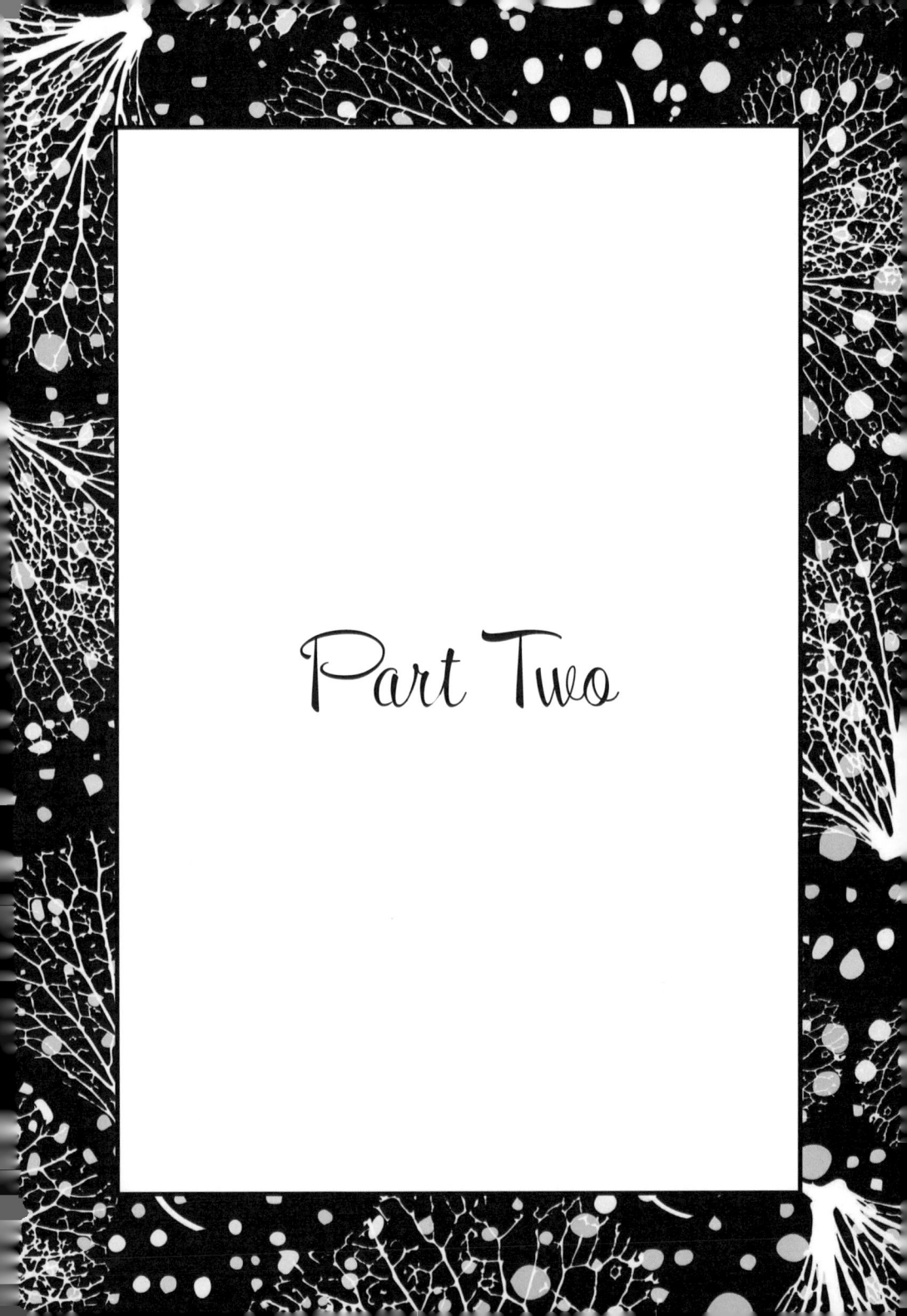

The journey continues...

I sincerely believe that knowledge is power, and when facing a health crisis, it is essential to become your own best health advocate. The principal way to do this, in my opinion, is to find out all you can about how a healthy heart works and to learn as much of the medical terminology as possible. This will place you in a stronger position to understand what you are being told and the ability to ask about your care from a more informed standpoint. Consequently, each medical appointment is likely to be more rewarding and allow you to ask pertinent questions about test results and treatment options.

Moreover, I have written this section, not only to help patients, but also to help those in a supporting role to garner a better understanding of the illnesses and ways in which they may help the patient. As you might imagine, the heart is a very complex and detailed subject. Therefore, I have tried to summarise the information for readers in a clear and concise format, occasionally including anecdotes to make it more personal and interesting to read.

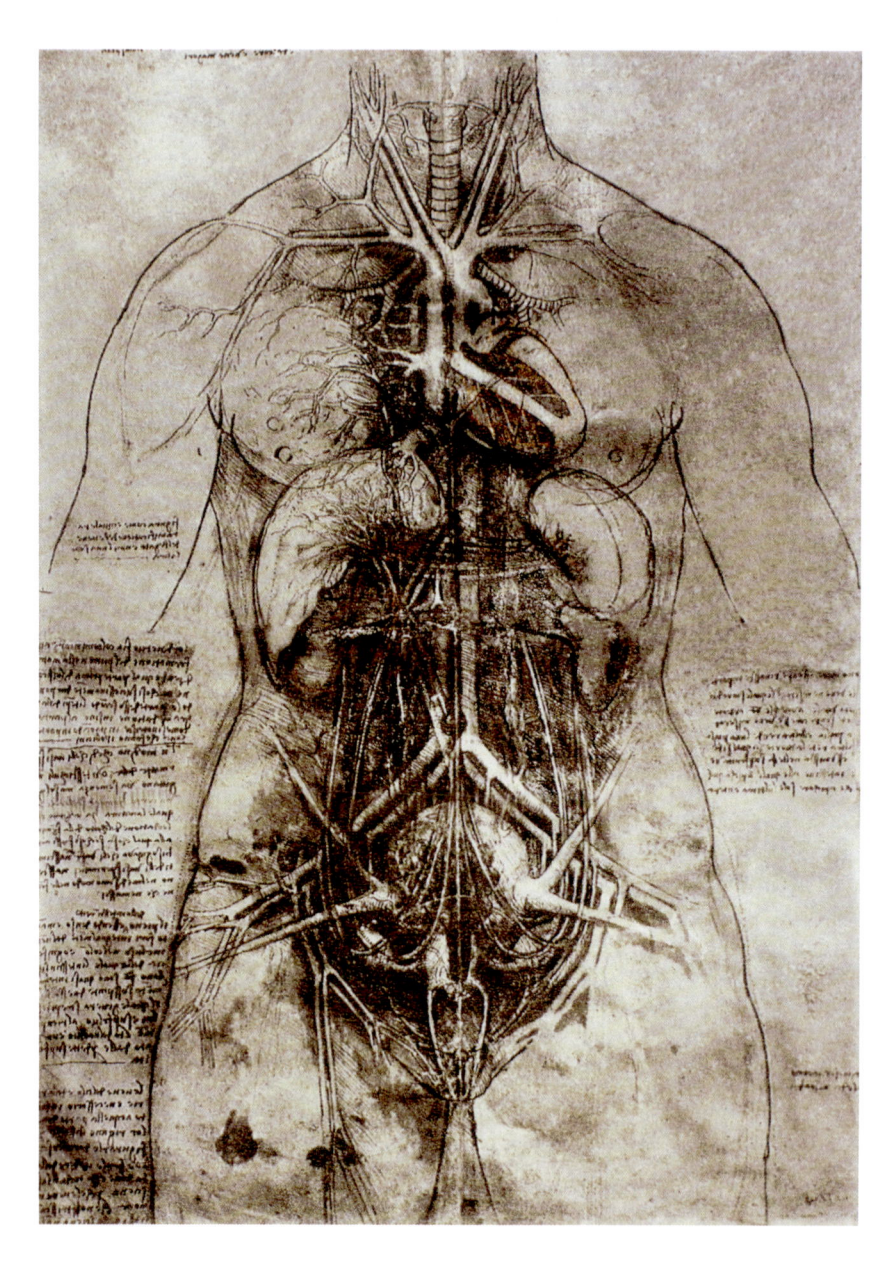

Credit: Science Photo Library

CHAPTER 18

"Tears come from the heart and not from the brain."

Leonardo da Vinci

Although Leonardo da Vinci was born in 1452 and died in 1519, just over 500 years ago, he made the most wonderful discoveries about the heart and produced beautiful, intricate, and sensitive drawings of its anatomy. In fact, many of his theories have only been validated in recent times. An Italian polymath of the Renaissance, Leonardo's areas of interest were drawing, painting, sculpture, invention, architecture, science, music, mathematics, engineering, literature, anatomy, geology, astronomy, botany, palaeontology, and cartography. This broad skillset gave him the unique ability to investigate and understand the workings of the heart as well as to capture its inherent beauty through his drawings.

I recently found a very interesting book called *The Heart of Leonardo* written by Francis Wells, a consultant cardiothoracic surgeon at Papworth Hospital in Cambridge, who has explored the vast wealth of information provided by Leonardo da Vinci and it contains many of Leonardo's beautiful drawings. It is fascinating to discover that someone of such great talent and curiosity paved the way for further understanding but rather unfortunate that these observations were not published during his lifetime and that sadly many of his notes and drawings, if not lost, remained undiscovered for some 200 years after his death.

Leonardo da Vinci was certainly well ahead of his time and his genius was demonstrated in his ability to study the heart in such depth by combining his knowledge of science, anatomy, engineering, and art. Performing multiple experiments on mammalian and human hearts, he realised that every heart contained a very clever piece of evolutionary engineering, three small pouches which sit directly above the aortic valve, and which are now called the sinuses of Valsalva. In fact, they ought to be called the sinuses of da Vinci because although they were named after the Italian anatomist, Antonio Valsalva, who published his findings, they had originally been discovered by Leonardo in 1513, some 200 years earlier.

Leonardo came to this conclusion while observing the eddies formed when water is forced through a small opening. He predicted that the ejected blood would possess 'revolving impetus' which would actively shut the aortic valve before the blood could flow backwards. He believed that the shape of the sinuses of Valsalva was formed deliberately in this way to create vortices to ensure synchronous, homogeneous, and stress-free leaflet closure with no regurgitation. He built a glass model of the aortic root with a porcine aortic valve at the base and pumped water through it containing grass seed, so that he could visualise and study the flow dynamics. Today's state of the art equipment, the 4-D flow MRI, clearly shows this theory to be correct, something Leonardo da Vinci had ingeniously discovered some 500 years ago without having access to today's advanced technologies.

The Complexities of the Heart...

The biggest heart that we know of is that of the blue whale. It weighs 400lb and is about the size of a small piano.

Whilst on a deep dive for food the blue whale lowers its heart rate to as little as two beats per minute and when it comes back to the surface to recover and reoxygenate its body, its heart rate returns to around 37 beats per minute. Its resting heart rate is only four to ten beats per minute.

The fastest heart rate is that of a pygmy shrew which beats at 1200–1500 beats per minute. In contrast, the human resting heart beats on average between 60–80 beats per minute, increasing to approximately 140 beats per minute while exercising.

As we grow older, the resting heart rate usually increases, and the heart rate is often lower in people who are physically fit.

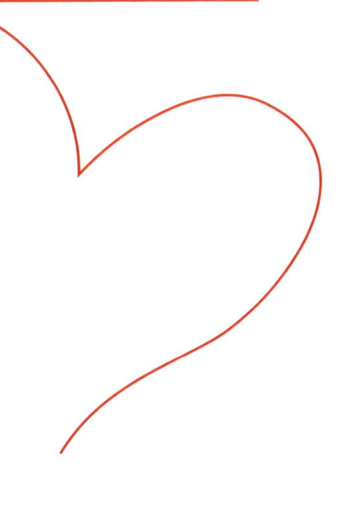

The Physical Heart...

The human heart is a hollow muscular organ located slightly to the left in the thoracic cavity and, whilst a single organ, it works as a double pump driving blood along two separate pathways in the circulatory system. With each beat, the heart's right ventricle pumps oxygen-depleted blood to the lungs to pick up oxygen and unload carbon dioxide, while the left ventricle simultaneously pumps the oxygenated blood from the lungs to cells throughout the entire body. Each full circulation takes only one minute.

The adult human heart is around the size of a fist and consists of four chambers, the right and left atrium, and the right and left ventricle. 'Atrium' is the Latin word for 'entrance hall', and 'ventricle' comes from the Latin, *ventriculus cordis*, meaning 'little pouch or little belly'. The heart is divided lengthwise by the septum which prevents oxygen-rich blood from mixing with oxygen-poor blood. It has four valves, tricuspid, mitral, aortic, and pulmonary. Each valve has three leaflets or cusps, except for the mitral valve which has just two.

The left ventricle is the stronger of the two ventricles and performs the more demanding part of the double-pump work. It has a thick muscular wall in comparison to the right ventricle whose wall is much thinner. In addition to moving oxygen throughout the body, the heart also helps deliver nutrients and picks up waste products. It beats three billion times in an average lifetime propelling approximately 200 million litres of blood. It takes a brief pause in between each beat but otherwise beats from the beginning to the end of one's life.

> ## The heart consists of several layers:
>
> - **The pericardium:** the outer fibrous sac offers a level of physical protection and helps to prevent the heart from overexpanding. The pericardium contains the coronary arteries which extend over the surface of the heart keeping it replenished with freshly oxygenated blood.
> - **The myocardium:** the strong muscular walls of the left and right atria, the left and right ventricles as well as the septum, contains bands of a specialised muscle called cardiac striated muscle which allows the heart to contract in the optimal way.
> - **The endocardium:** a thin inner layer of the heart consisting of squamous vascular endothelial cells, which ensures that the blood flows smoothly inside the heart and reduces turbulence.

Blood flow is regulated by the four valves, and these are cleverly designed to ensure a one-way flow. However, these valves are not actively contracting but opening and closing because of pressure changes developed by the contraction of the heart. The aortic valve is further assisted in this process by the presence of the sinuses of Valsalva which help to ensure its efficient closure. The valves are supported by tendinous cords (chordae tendineae) which prevent the valves from opening in the opposite direction and are rooted into the wall of the heart via the papillary muscles.

At the beginning of the cardiac cycle, while the atria and ventricles are relaxed, blood flows from the vena cava into the right atrium and from the four pulmonary veins into the left atrium before flowing uninterrupted through the open tricuspid valve on the right and the mitral valve on the left into the ventricles below. This process is called diastole. The ventricles fill with blood at a steadily decreasing rate until the pressure in the ventricles is equal to that in the veins. At the end of diastole, when approximately two thirds of the blood has entered the ventricles, the atria contract, known as an atrial kick, forcing the remaining one third of blood into the ventricles. This increases the pressure within the ventricles so that it is now higher than that in the atria causing the atrioventricular (tricuspid and mitral) valves to shut producing a sound known as 'Lub'.

During the next phase both sets of valves are closed so that no blood can escape from the ventricles. As soon as the pressure in the ventricles exceeds the pressure in the pulmonary artery and aorta, the pulmonary and aortic valves open and blood is pumped from the heart into the great arteries. This phase of the cardiac cycle is called systole. At the end of systole, the ventricles begin to relax and this decrease in pressure compared to the aorta and the pulmonary artery causes the valves to shut, producing a sound known as 'Dub'. This explains the familiar sound of a normal heartbeat heard through a stethoscope – Lub-Dub, Lub-Dub, Lub-Dub.

The contraction of the heart is like wringing water out a towel. This motion is called a cardiac twist, where the cardiac contraction goes inwards, upwards, and twists. The shape of the heart is designed to encourage this motion and makes the heart more efficient.

As you can see from the table below, the pressures in the left heart are much higher than those in the right heart. This is because the left ventricle needs to pump the oxygenated blood throughout the whole body, from the top of the head to the tips of the toes, whereas the right ventricle only needs to pump the deoxygenated blood to the lungs, a much shorter distance. This would also explain why the sinuses of Valsalva are only found in the aortic root as the aorta must endure much higher pressures. Furthermore, the ascending portion of the aorta is where the origin of the right and left coronary arteries resides. They exit the ascending aorta immediately above the aortic valve at the sinuses of Valsalva. Blood flow into these arteries is greatest during ventricular diastole when aortic pressure is at its peak and greater than the pressure in the coronaries.

Pressures within the heart

Area of the heart	Pressure (mmHg)
Aorta	120 systolic; 80 diastolic
Left Atrium	8–10
Left Ventricle	120 systolic; 10 diastolic
Pulmonary Artery	25 systolic; 10 diastolic
Right Atrium	0–4
Right Ventricle	25 systolic; 4 diastolic

The Electrical Heart...

The impulse to stimulate cardiac contraction is intrinsic to the heart itself. In other words, if the brain were no longer to function and the nerves were interrupted, the heart would continue to beat independently as long as it had an adequate supply of oxygen. This electrical signal can be recorded by placing electrodes on the chest and is called an electrocardiogram (ECG, or EKG). It was invented in 1903 by Dutch physiologist Willem Einthoven and is still used to diagnose cardiac problems to this day. The importance of his discovery was recognised by his award of the Nobel Prize for Physiology of Medicine in 1924, and there is no doubt that his discovery was momentous and helped to provide a window into the electrical conductivity of the heart.

The cardiac electrical signal controls the heartbeat in two ways. Firstly, since each electrical impulse generates one heartbeat, the number of electrical impulses determines the heart rate. Secondly, as the electrical signal spreads across the heart, it triggers the heart muscle to contract in the correct sequence, thus coordinating each heartbeat and assuring that the heart works as efficiently as possible.

The heart's electrical signal is produced by a tiny structure known as the sinus node (SN), which is located in the upper portion of the right atrium.

From the sinus node, the electrical signal spreads across the right and left atria causing them both to contract, and to push their load of blood into the right and left ventricles. The electrical signal then passes through the atrioventricular node (AV node) to the ventricles, where it causes the ventricles to contract.

Separating the atria from the ventricles is a fibrous 'disc' called the AV disc, and this cleverly prevents the passage of the electrical signal between the atria and the ventricles. Consequently, the only way the signal can get from the atria to the ventricles is through the AV node and this avoids any errant messages pacing the heart at the wrong time.

Cardiac muscle cells are able to contract on their own but without the correct pacing from the sinus node different muscle cells would beat at different rates, e.g., the atria cells beat more rapidly than those in the ventricles. Without the unity of the overriding signal from the sinus node the heart would be inefficient and pump in an uncoordinated manner.

Heart rate is modified by the parasympathetic and sympathetic branches of the autonomic nervous system (ANS). Parasympathetic activity is mediated via acetylcholine acting on receptors at the SA node, slowing the heart rate. Sympathetic activity is mediated via noradrenaline increasing the heart rate. The average resting heart rate of 60 beats per minute (bpm) is dominated by the parasympathetic system at rest, and increased sympathetic outflow increases bpm accordingly. However, if all autonomic inputs to the heart are blocked, the intrinsic heart rate is about 100bpm as in the case of heart transplant recipients whose nerves have been severed.

Most cardiac arrests occur when a heart's electrical system malfunctions. This malfunction causes an abnormal heart rhythm such as ventricular tachycardia or ventricular fibrillation. Some cardiac arrests are also caused by extreme slowing of the heart's rhythm called bradycardia.

Further heart rhythm disorders caused by problems in the heart's electrical system include atrial fibrillation and atrial flutter. Atrial fibrillation is a common disorder that causes the heart to beat in abnormal patterns. In atrial flutter, the atria beat too rapidly but the heart rhythm is more organised and less chaotic than that of atrial fibrillation. Sometimes, these errant electrical impulses may reach the ventricles and cause them to contract faster and less efficiently than normal.

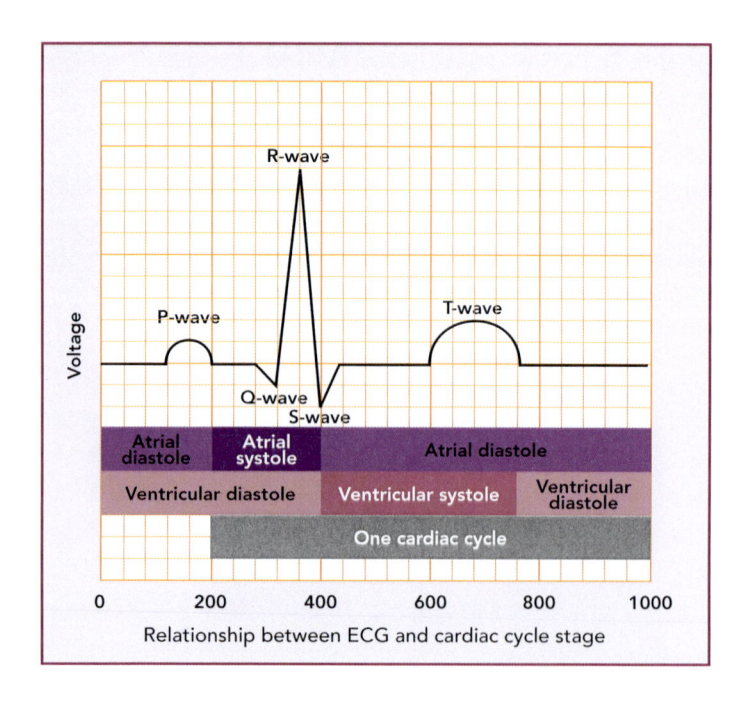

Relationship between ECG and cardiac cycle stage

> ## *The Calmer Heart...*
>
> An extremely important player in slowing the heart rate is the 'vagus' nerve which carries an extensive range of signals from the brain, heart, lungs, and digestive tract and vice versa. Although referred to as a single nerve, it comes as a pair, one for the right and one for the left side of the body and is the longest and most important nerve in the human body. The origin of the word 'vagus' comes from the Latin for 'wandering' as it weaves its way throughout the body. It is believed that the vagus nerve is responsible for the 'mind–body' connection and activation of this nerve results in the calming of bodily functions, including slowing of the heart rate.

There are times when the parasympathetic system may become overstimulated, as in the case of high-endurance athletes. Their vagal tone may be so elevated that their heart rate may slow excessively to a level where the sinus node is unable to override the other impulses within the heart. This in turn can lead to premature atrial contractions, atrial fibrillation, paroxysmal a-fib and other arrhythmias.

In general terms, if the heart is damaged or structurally abnormal, arrhythmias are more likely to be sympathetically mediated. On the other hand, if the heart is structurally sound, it is more likely that any arrhythmias may be parasympathetically mediated.

Abnormalities in the heart's electrical system can lead to problems with the heart rate being too fast or too slow or can entirely disrupt the normal functioning of the heart, even if the heart's muscles and valves themselves are entirely normal.

The Valsalva manoeuvre is an internationally recognised technique, under medical supervision, which can be used to help restore a normal heart rate in patients with supraventricular tachycardia. Named after 17th century Italian physician Antonio Maria Valsalva (see also sinuses of Valsalva pages 162 and 167), the Valsalva manoeuvre (VM) changes the pressure within the chest and abdomen and causes the body to try to compensate for the increased pressure by slowing the heart. This is done by breathing forcefully against a closed airway for fifteen seconds, blocking expiratory air from leaving the body via the mouth and nose. The Valsalva manoeuvre is also sometimes used to diagnose heart conditions or problems with the autonomic nervous system.

The Gastric Heart...

Many people may suffer with a condition known as 'gastrocardiac syndrome' and this may even occur when the heart is not damaged. Some of these symptoms may include burping, nausea, heartburn, palpitations, and changes in blood pressure. There are several reasons why the stomach and oesophagus may give cardiac symptoms and vice versa:

- Anatomically, the oesophagus, stomach, and heart are in very close proximity and are supplied by the same nerve, the vagus nerve.
- Medications may impact the digestion, e.g., proton pump inhibitors (PPIs) inhibit acid in the stomach and may lead to reduced absorption of vital nutrients, in particular magnesium, which may lead to ectopic heart beats (PVCs).
- Reflux (GERD), dyspepsia as well as chronic inflammation can all trigger palpitations. Furthermore, hiatus hernia and a full or distended stomach may push against the diaphragm impinging on the heart and causing it to change position which in turn may trigger PVCs and/or palpitations.
- Sleeping position may also affect the vagus nerve and some studies show that lying on the right-hand side may have more of an impact on the vagus nerve than lying on the left or on the back.
- Some of these symptoms may also be present in the instance of myocarditis, see Chapter 19 for details.

> ## *The Damaged Heart Muscle...*
>
> Most people have the good fortune to start out in life with a pristine heart, just like a brand-new piece of paper. Drawing on that paper with ink is an irrevocable act, just as folding the paper has a similar irreversibility. Likewise, any damage to the heart leaves an indelible mark, and despite years of research it has never been possible to recover the heart to its original state.

Unfortunately, the heart muscle does not repair itself very effectively. When damaged, the left ventricle often becomes less flexible and fibrotic, and the stiffness prevents the heart from pumping to its full capacity. The right ventricle, on the other hand, may become thin, dilated and less able to contract effectively. Cardiac myocytes (the cells of the myocardium) have their own rhythm and continue to cycle within a normal timeframe; they do not know they are damaged and now require longer to contract and dilate. As a result, a scarred heart will no longer get a full contraction or dilation making it weak and the individual easily tired. If the heart has dilated, the valves may be overstretched preventing the leaflets from closing properly and this allows a back flow of blood into the atria, called regurgitation.

Of course, when you are in good health, you are not usually aware of your heart beating inside your chest, except when exercising or feeling anxious, and take for granted that your heart will always adapt to your ongoing requirements. Unfortunately, if the heart has been damaged, there is likely to be much less reserve. This is particularly important when crossing a busy road. In the past I would have just run across, but now I make sure I have enough time to cross without causing a strain. With heart failure, it takes much longer for the arteries to dilate fully and adapt to the extra requirements placed upon them. Consequently, a very gradual increase in speed at the beginning of an exercise session will allow for this adaptation to take place and enable you to continue at a good pace for much longer without stopping. I have also learnt that strong calf muscles play an important role in helping the heart to circulate the blood whilst walking.

Stop exercising and consider calling your healthcare provider if you experience any of the following warning symptoms:

- Pressure or pain in your chest, neck, arm, jaw, or shoulder
- Dizziness or lightheadedness
- Nausea
- Unusual shortness of breath
- Unusual tiredness
- Fast or slow heartbeat
- Irregular heartbeat

Source: Intermountain Healthcare – Living with Heart Failure

The Metaphorical Heart...

Another part of the wondrous heart is what I would call the 'metaphorical heart'. There is such a rich history of expressions describing the heart in this way and throughout the world the heart continues to be a symbol of emotion for all human beings. The plethora of heart metaphors wonderfully captures the heart's emotions – happiness, sadness, elation, grief, wonderment, sorrow, excitement, disappointment, shock, and fear, and I have provided you with some examples on the page opposite.

Heart Throb
Eat your heart out
Have heart stand still
From the bottom of your heart
Pure of Heart
Have a heart to heart
Change of Heart
To give someone heart failure
HAVE ONES BEST INTEREST AT HEART
Heart sinks
Cross my heart
heart goes out
Young at heart
Heart of the matter
Heart skips a beat
Heart of Stone
Grateful Heart
Faint Heart
Smiling heart
SPEAKING FROM THE HEART
Wearing your heart on your sleeve
Darling Heart
Heart of Gold
Learning by Heart
Broken Heart
WOUNDED HEART
Leaping heart
Way to a man's heart is through his stomach
Lion Heart
Forgiving Heart
Heart Melting
Have one's heart in the right place
Heart sinks

The Electrolyte Heart...

A finely tuned balance of electrolytes in the blood, such as potassium, sodium, calcium, magnesium, phosphorus, chloride and bicarbonate, is essential to the proper functioning of the heart. Electrolytes are responsible for several important functions. In addition to regulating fluids, they also transmit nerve signals from the heart, muscles, and nerve cells to other cells; they help in the building of new tissue; support blood clotting; they keep the beating of the heart by electrically stimulating muscle contractions; maintain the blood's pH level and regulate the fluid level in blood plasma.

Therefore, an imbalance of electrolytes can affect the heart's electrical impulses and contribute to arrhythmia development. Additionally, certain medications will have a direct effect on the balance of electrolytes in the blood, and it is essential to learn the warning signs of a possible excess or deficiency in any of these elements (see Chapter 20).

> ## *The Sensitive Heart...*
>
> Having experienced such a rare and intense assault on my heart, I feel that I am unusually placed to appreciate that the heart is wonderfully complex. Its function appears to be influenced by so many different elements, and modern medicine does not always take these into account. As I was attached to a heart monitor continuously for seven weeks, it was particularly interesting for me to observe the multiple factors which influenced my heart function. The impact of each factor was often amplified by the fragility and susceptibility of my own damaged heart.

If you were to ask someone how they feel when they lose a loved one, most would say they feel it in their heart. In fact, there is even an illness which may arise following an emotional shock called 'broken-heart syndrome' or 'takotsubo' when the heart swells and suddenly develops cardiomyopathy. This may explain why, in the elderly population some husbands and wives die very soon after their spouse – they literally die of a broken heart.

While many in the scientific community are still doggedly attached to the concept of the heart as being solely a mechanical pump influenced by the brain and nothing more, some researchers are now beginning to explore the possibility that the heart may have its own brain.

This concept may seem rather farfetched, but Professor David Paterson, Professor of Cardiovascular

Physiology at Oxford University, who leads a research team in cardiac neurobiology, has delved into the intricacies of the heart and discovered that the brain is not the sole source of emotions but indeed the heart and brain work together in producing emotions. He has discovered that the right ventricle of the heart contains a network of thousands of specialised neurons. Neurons are what allow the brain to form thoughts, and Professor Paterson has demonstrated through experiments with heart tissue that the 'brain' in the heart communicates back and forth with the brain in the head. It's a two-way street. This discovery would therefore appear to confirm what many have always believed, that the heart is indeed the seat of all emotions and that this hypothesis may have been correct after all.

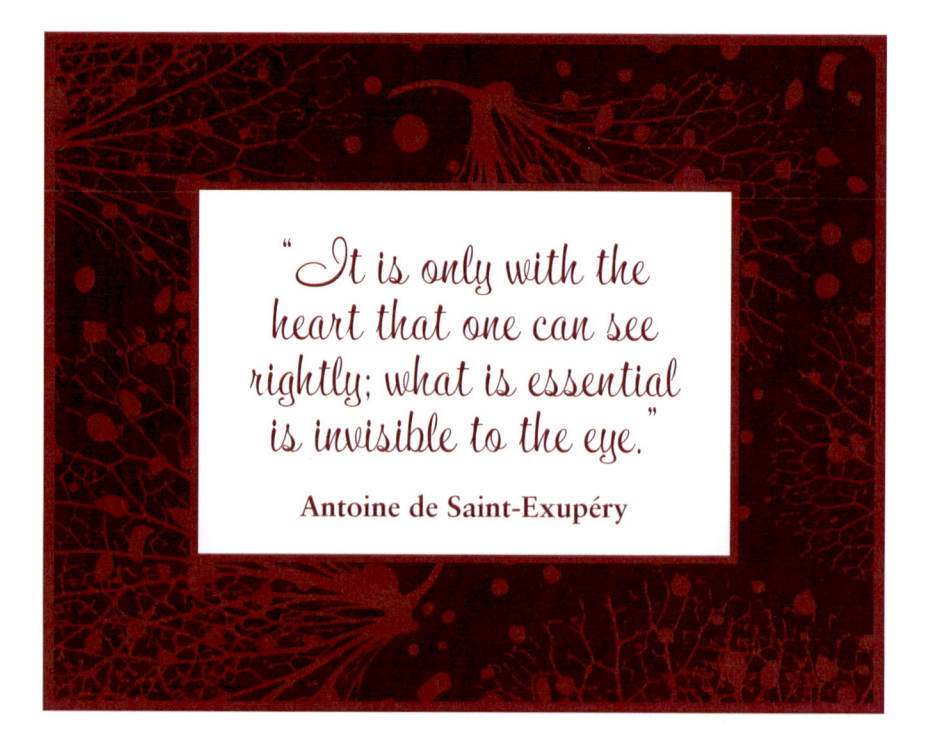

> "It is only with the heart that one can see rightly; what is essential is invisible to the eye."
>
> **Antoine de Saint-Exupéry**

> ## *The Future...*
>
> There are a multitude of therapies and cardiac tests which are now available to help cardiac patients monitor, regain, and maintain cardiac function. The more successful are usually in the field of interventional cardiology, including stents, bypass surgery, valve replacements, implantable cardioverter defibrillators (ICDs), pacemakers and even heart transplants.
>
> Interventionist cardiology is now moving forward in leaps and bounds, and there are even wireless pacemakers which may be inserted during a cath procedure. The device is ten times smaller than a conventional pacemaker and relies on a built-in battery which lasts between 9 and 13 years. Inserted through a catheter, it is designed to be easily retrievable, so that it can be replaced with minimal surgery.

It is my hope that at some point heart failure cardiology will eventually catch up. However, the reality is that there has been little progress in cardiac muscle disease treatment in the past 20 years despite the best medical efforts. The usual treatment being cardiac medication, reduced salt, reduced fluids, behaviour modification and in severe cases left ventricular assist devices, the Impella heart pump and heart transplantation.

In the case of cardiac muscle disease there is now a new cardiac blood test, called the 'ST2' cardiac function test, which is available in the USA but, at the time of writing this book, not currently in the UK. 'ST2' signals the presence and severity of adverse cardiac remodelling and tissue fibrosis which occurs in response to myocardial infarction, acute coronary syndrome, or worsening heart failure. There are, of course, two other essential blood tests 'High Sensitivity Troponin T' and 'NT-proBNP' which are now the gold standard.

Stem cell research is ongoing. The theory is to use the patient's own stem cells to promote the regeneration of heart muscle and blood vessel cells. Stem cells may be derived from the patient's bone marrow or heart tissue. This treatment is not yet in the mainstream and work continues to be carried out to demonstrate the efficacy and safety of these treatments.

Further research is also being carried out to investigate regeneration of the cardiac myocytes from studies looking at the zebrafish: a fish that is uniquely able to regenerate its own heart. Researchers are also looking at the possibility of switching on the 'MYC' gene together with the 'CCNT1' gene to allow the heart to regenerate and then to be able to switch them off again.

Unfortunately, in my own experience, whilst new treatments are frequently mentioned in the media, access to them is invariably limited to clinical trials, many doctors may not be aware of these treatments and it may be a decade before they become mainstream, if at all.

I have not stopped looking for a solution to my heart condition and I continue to work tirelessly to understand what impacts my heart and body in positive and negative ways so that I may adjust accordingly. You may also be interested in reading about several lifestyle changes which I have adopted, and which have helped me to stay on top of my illness (see Chapters 20 to 24).

One of the founders of the Mayo Clinic, William J. Mayo, once said that 'A specialist is someone who knows more and more about less and less, until they know everything about nothing.' I can't help thinking that by following the example of Leonardo da Vinci, a more comprehensive understanding of all elements of the heart within the context of the human body, a multi-disciplinary approach, might just help us to find further cures, rather than fixing each piece individually like a mechanic approaches a car repair.

CHAPTER 19

"A good head and a good heart are always a formidable combination."

Nelson Mandela

Many people have never heard of myocarditis, perhaps a few more have heard of cardiomyopathy and probably considerably more have heard of heart failure. However, the latter is often misunderstood, and some imagine that heart failure implies that the heart is just about to stop.

When I first received my diagnosis, I started to do extensive research and was surprised to learn that several famous people have died of the above illnesses. Unfortunately, however, despite their renown, overall knowledge of these diseases remains extremely patchy.

One of my favourite singers, George Michael, sadly died suddenly of myocarditis and cardiomyopathy at the age of 53 in 2016; Andy Gibb, younger brother of the Bee Gees, died of myocarditis at the age of 30; another talented singer, Natalie Cole, died of congestive heart failure at the age of 65; Miles Frost, son of Sir David Frost, died of hypertrophic cardiomyopathy suddenly at the age of 31; and plastic surgeon, Dr. Martin Kelly, died suddenly of cardiomyopathy at the age of 43. In many of these cases it appears they were totally unaware of any cardiac issues.

What is Myocarditis?
(myo=muscle; cardi=heart; itis=inflammation)

> **Myocarditis is a disease marked by inflammation and damage to the heart muscle. It usually attacks otherwise healthy people and can be the cause of sudden death. As mentioned previously, the cases of myocarditis and associated cardiomyopathy have increased over the last few decades.**

There are multiple types of myocarditis including fulminant, giant cell, eosinophilic, lymphocytic, autoimmune, viral, bacterial, immunologic and physical. It is often believed that myocarditis is a rare disease. The incidence and prevalence of myocarditis are not known from population-based studies because there is no widely available test that can be applied at a population level. However, although the exact incidence of myocarditis is not known, it was estimated that there were approximately 3.1 million cases of myocarditis worldwide in 2017. Furthermore, it is thought that up to 20% of sudden death cases in young adults have been reported to be due to myocarditis.

Many of the causes of myocarditis are listed in the table opposite. As you can see, there are so many possible causes that diagnosis is often protracted and sometimes the underlying aetiology may never be found. Whilst many cases of myocarditis are self-resolving some develop chronic inflammatory myocarditis (as in my case) which is more difficult to manage. Inflammation, whilst

INFECTIOUS CAUSES

Viral Agents
- Adenoviruses
- Arboviruses
- Cytomegaloviruses
- Enteroviruses (coxsackie B)
- Herpes viruses (human herpes virus 6; Epstein–Barr)
- Hepatitis C virus
- HIV-1
- Influenza A
- Mumps
- Parvovirus B-19
- Poliomyelitis
- Rabies
- Respiratory syncytial virus
- Rubeola
- SARS-CoV-2
- Varicella
- Variola/vaccinia
- Yellow fever virus

Spirochetal Agents
- Borrelia/Lyme disease
- Leptospirosis (Weil's disease)
- Syphilis

Rickettsial Agents
- Rocky Mountain spotted fever
- Scrub typhus
- Q fever

Fungal agents
- Actinomycosis
- Aspergillosis
- Blastomycosis
- Candidiasis
- Coccidioidomycosis
- Cryptococcosis
- Histoplasmosis
- Mucormycosis

Parasitic agents
- Cysticercosis
- Echinococcosis
- Filariasis
- Heterophyiasis
- Schistosomiasis
- Trichinosis
- Visceral larva migrans

Bacterial agents
- Borrelia species
- Brucellosis
- Clostridia
- Diphtheria
- Melioidosis
- Meningococci
- Mycobacterium species
- Mycoplasma pneumoniae
- Psittacosis
- Staphylococci
- Streptococci
- Treponema pallidum
- Tuberculosis

Protozoal agents
- Balantidiasis
- Leishmaniasis
- Malaria
- Sarcosporidiosis
- Toxoplasmosis
- Trypanosoma cruzi (Chagas disease)
- Trypanosomiasis

NON-INFECTIOUS CAUSES

Systemic inflammatory diseases
- Acute rheumatic fever
- Crohn's disease
- Churg–Strauss syndrome
- Diabetes mellitus
- Giant cell myocarditis
- Kawasaki disease
- Rheumatoid arthritis
- Sarcoidosis
- Scleroderma
- Systemic lupus erythematosus
- Takayasu arteritis
- Thyrotoxicosis
- Ulcerative colitis
- Wegener granulomatosis
- Thyrotoxicosis

Physical agents
- Heatstroke
- Hypothermia
- Radiation

Hypersensitivity
- Antibiotics: penicillin, cephalosporins, chloramphenicol, sulfonamides
- Antihypertensive drugs: methyldopa, spironolactone
- Antiseizure drugs: phenytoin, carbamazepine
- Digoxin
- Diuretics
- Dobutamine
- Tricyclic antidepressants

Chemical Agents
- Arsenic
- Carbon monoxide
- Cobalt
- Hydrocarbons
- Lead
- Mercury
- Phosphorus

Toxins
- Drugs: amphetamines, cocaine, catecholamines
- Chemotherapeutic drugs: doxorubicin and anthracyclines, streptomycin, cyclophosphamide, interleukin-2, anti-HER-2 receptor antibody/Herceptin
- Vaccines: Covid-19; smallpox

Bites/stings
- Black widow spider venom
- Scorpion venom
- Snake venom
- Tick paralysis
- Wasp venom

Other
- Peripartum cardiomyopathy
- Post-transplant cellular rejection

important for acute conditions like a broken ankle, is harmful if the inflammation continues unabated, as in the case of autoimmune myocarditis, it ends up damaging healthy cardiac tissue.

Additionally, some of the new treatments for cancer may cause a very rare form of myocarditis. It is also to be noted that most recently SARS-CoV-2 has also been shown in some cases to infiltrate the heart and to cause myocarditis. Furthermore, patients that have recovered from SARS-CoV-2 can be left with some residual heart damage and cardiac problems.

Although myocarditis may seem relatively rare, it often leads to dilated cardiomyopathy and heart failure. Expert consensus opinion estimates that up to 40% of dilated cardiomyopathy results from myocarditis. Often, particularly in the milder cases of the disease, people may be unaware they have suffered with myocarditis only to find out later as their heart function begins to deteriorate. Therefore, I believe, it is essential for people to be able to recognise the diverse symptoms of myocarditis and hopefully save lives from greater awareness (see table opposite).

For those suffering with myocarditis, the prognosis is variable but chronic heart failure is a frequent major long-term complication. Myocarditis and the associated disorder of idiopathic dilated cardiomyopathy are the cause of approximately 45% of heart transplants in the United States.

Symptoms of Myocarditis

I have compiled the following list and have personally experienced all of these symptoms. However, some people may only experience a small number making myocarditis difficult to diagnose. Therefore, in my opinion, if you or your doctor observe any of these warning signs (in no particular order), further investigations including a troponin T and NT-proBNP blood test and an echo may prove to be lifesaving.

- Shortness of breath
- Tachycardia (increased heart rate)
- Pain in the chest/shoulder/arm/ribs on the left-hand side/discomfort in raising the arms above the head
- Fever
- Frequent eructation (burping), sudden onset and unusual
- Perspiration, particularly across the abdomen and neck
- A feeling of cold clamminess across the skin
- Ectopic heartbeats
- Irritability, anxiety and an inability to feel settled
- Prominent jugular veins
- 3rd heart sound
- Poor circulation
- Grey pallor
- Tickling sensation within the left side of the chest

Diagnosis:

Accurate diagnosis of myocarditis requires a cardiac biopsy or autopsy (if the patient has died). However, when this invasive method is not possible, clinical observations of probable acute myocarditis may be extrapolated from the following:
- Heart failure of less than 3 months
- Unexplained elevation in troponin T blood test
- Normal coronary arteries
- ECG features of myocardial injury
- New wall motion abnormality
- Pericardial effusion on echo
- Characteristic tissue features on MRI

Treatment:

Standard treatment of myocarditis involves:
- Cardiac rest to ease the heart's workload
- Standard heart failure therapy (medication and lifestyle changes, including fluid and salt reduction)
- Immunomodulating and immuno-suppressive therapies for chronic and virus negative inflammation
- Avoidance of competitive sports for 3–6 months
- Frequent monitoring with exercise tests, ECG, echos, Holter monitoring, and MRI
- Implantable cardiac defibrillators, if required
- Cardiac transplant, in severe cases

What is Cardiomyopathy? (BHF)
(cardio=heart; myo=muscle; pathy=disease)

> **Cardiomyopathy is a progressive disease of the heart muscle which affects its size, shape, and structure. The more common cardiomyopathies include hypertrophic cardiomyopathy and dilated cardiomyopathy.**

Cardiomyopathy is often inherited. Some members of a family may be affected more than others and some family members may not be affected or have any symptoms.

It is estimated that 750,000 people in the United States have dilated cardiomyopathy and that roughly half of these cases are familial. 40% of cases are thought to be associated with inflammation by a previous or current viral infection.

One in 500 people in the United States are estimated to have hypertrophic cardiomyopathy and may not know they have the condition. Cardiomyopathy is a leading cause of heart failure and the most common reason for needing a heart transplant.

> Cardiomyopathy is particularly dangerous because it often goes unrecognised and untreated.

Types of Cardiomyopathies

- Arrhythmogenic right ventricular cardiomyopathy (ARVC)
- Dilated cardiomyopathy (DCM)
- Hypertrophic cardiomyopathy (HCM)
- Takotsubo cardiomyopathy. This can be caused by extreme stress, is not passed on through families and often disappears over time.

Other, specialised types of cardiomyopathies include:

- Ischemic cardiomyopathy (IC)
- Ion channelopathies, eg the long QT syndrome and the very rare short QT syndrome
- Left ventricular non-compaction (LVNC)
- Peripartum cardiomyopathy (PPCM)
- Restrictive cardiomyopathy (RCM)

What is Heart Failure?

> **Heart failure, sometimes referred to as congestive heart failure, is caused by the heart being unable to pump effectively enough to maintain blood flow and fulfil all the body's needs.**

It is thought that approximately 5.8 million Americans have heart failure and that around 680,000 new cases are diagnosed every year. Moreover, heart failure is the number one reason for hospitalisations in individuals 65 years and older in the United Kingdom.

Heart failure is usually classified according to the severity of the patient's symptoms. The most commonly used description is the New York Heart Association Functional Classification and it has four categories:

Class	Patient Symptoms
I	No limitation of physical activity. Ordinary physical activity does not cause undue fatigue, palpitation, or dyspnea (shortness of breath).
II	Ordinary physical activity results in fatigue, palpitation and dyspnea (shortness of breath).
III	Marked limitation of physical activity. Comfortable at rest. Less than ordinary activity causes fatigue, palpitation, and dyspnea. Unable to carry on any physical activity without discomfort.
IV	Symptoms of heart failure at rest. If any physical activity is undertaken, discomfort increases.

Source: Intermountain Healthcare – Living with Heart Failure

UNDERSTANDING HEART FAILURE

UNDERSTANDING HEART FAILURE

Your treatment plan will make more sense to you if you have a good understanding of what happens when you have heart failure. But first, it helps to know how a healthy heart works.

HOW DOES A HEALTHY HEART WORK?

Your heart's job is to pump blood, rich in oxygen and nutrients, to all parts of your body. The figure below shows how this happens.

Your hard-working heart

Your heart is a hard-working muscle. On average, it beats 60 to 100 times each minute, every day of your life. Each beat pumps blood to all parts of your body.

By the time you're 70 years old, your heart will have pumped almost 50 million gallons of blood – quite a feat for an organ about the size of your fist!

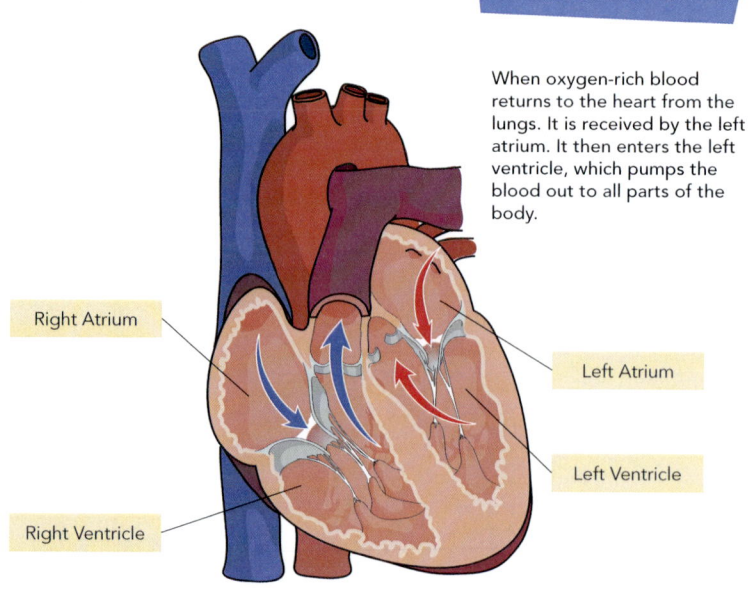

The four pumping chambers of the heart

Veins return oxygen-poor blood from the body to the right atrium of the heart. From there, the blood enters the right ventricle, which pumps the blood to the lungs to get a fresh supply of oxygen.

When oxygen-rich blood returns to the heart from the lungs. It is received by the left atrium. It then enters the left ventricle, which pumps the blood out to all parts of the body.

- Right Atrium
- Left Atrium
- Left Ventricle
- Right Ventricle

Source: Intermountain Healthcare – Living with Heart Failure

UNDERSTANDING HEART FAILURE

WHAT HAPPENS WITH HEART FAILURE?

When you have heart failure, your heart can't pump enough blood to meet your body's needs. This happens because your heart is weakened by conditions or diseases that damage the heart muscle. Most of these conditions weaken your heart little by little, over a period of time. Here's a summary of how heart failure can develop and progress.

1. The heart muscle is weakened by conditions or diseases that damage your heart.

2. The heart's pumping action becomes less efficient.

3. The body tries to compensate for the heart's reduced pumping action in these ways:
   - Hormonal stimulation to the heart increases.
   - The heart beats faster.
   - The heart enlarges. (Heart chambers stretch and get bigger, and the muscle mass may increase in size.)

4. For a time these adaptations will help continue normal or near-normal heart function. But sooner or later, these adjustments can actually make matters worse by putting extra strain on your heart.

5. Eventually the muscle will begin to wear out and become even less efficient at pumping the blood your body needs. Heart failure symptoms – such as shortness of breath, cough, fatigue, and fluid buildup – may begin or worsen.

Poor **squeeze** vs. poor **relaxation**

Heart failure occurs for two different reasons:

- Usually heart failure occurs because your heart isn't pumping effectively — you have "poor squeeze," or systolic heart failure.

- In some cases, the heart can still pump effectively — but the muscle walls have stiffened, which prevents the heart from fully relaxing and filling with enough blood between contractions.

This condition is called diastolic heart failure. With both types of heart failure, your heart can't deliver enough blood to your body. This can interfere with the function of other major organs, and produce a range of symptoms throughout your body.

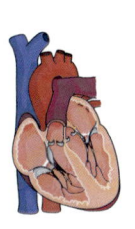

---

normal heart

initial damage
weakness heart muscle

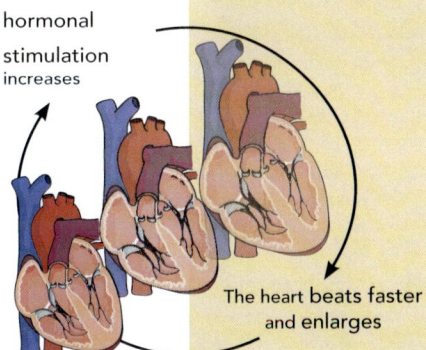

to compensate...

hormonal stimulation increases

The heart beats faster and enlarges

heart muscle begins to wear out

195

Source: Intermountain Healthcare – Living with Heart Failure

UNDERSTANDING HEART FAILURE

WHAT ARE THE SYMPTOMS OF HEART FAILURE?

Your heart failure symptoms are due to either fluid buildup or lack of oxygen in your tissues. You may notice some – or all – of these heart failure symptoms:

- Shortness of breath. You may experience shortness of breath at any time. This is due to the fluid buildup in your lungs, which makes breathing harder. This breathing difficulty tends to occur first during physical activity – and may also occur at night when you're lying flat.

- Cough. Many people with heart failure complain of a frequent cough. Sometimes this cough is dry and hacking, and other times it produces phlegm. For some, this cough occurs primarily at night. For others, it can last all day. Like shortness of breath, this cough is likely a side effect of fluid buildup in your lungs, especially if your phlegm is pink-tinged.

- Excessive fatigue. When your heart can't pump enough blood to meet your body's needs, you're bound to feel more tired than usual. You may also feel weak. Your muscles and organs simply aren't getting the blood they need, and even a good night's sleep won't help.

- Weight gain. Weight gain may be one of the earliest signs of fluid buildup in your body. Extra fluid in your body translates into extra weight showing up on your scale – at a rate of about 2 pounds for each quart of additional body fluid. For this reason, keeping track of your weight is an important measure of your heart failure management.

- Swollen ankles, feet, belly, lower back and fingers. Fluid buildup will show up as swelling in different parts of your body. The ankles, feet, belly, lower back and fingers are places where extra fluid is most likely to collect as it seeps out of the blood vessels into your tissues. Swelling in your belly can cause you to feel bloated or nauseated, and can decrease your appetite. Swelling is usually worse at the end of the day.

- Poor concentration and memory lapses. Some people with heart failure complain of difficulty concentrating and lapses in memory. These symptoms may be explained by less oxygen being delivered to the brain.

You could have right-sided heart failure, left-sided heart failure – or both

Right-sided heart failure

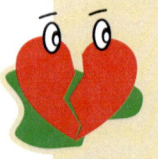

When the right side of the heart isn't pumping effectively, the blood returning to the heart from the body backs up in the veins. When blood backs up in the veins, excess fluid in the blood leaks out into the surrounding tissues. This can cause:

- Swelling in the liver
- Bloating in the stomach
- Swelling in the legs and ankles.

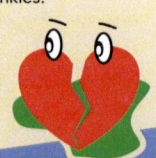

Left-sided heart failure

When the left side of the heart isn't pumping effectively, blood backs up, causing fluid accumulation in the lungs. This can cause:

- Shortness of breath
- Cough
- Fatigue and weakness

Source: Intermountain Healthcare – Living with Heart Failure

LIFESTYLE MANAGEMENT

LIFESTYLE MANAGEMENT

Managing heart failure means creating and following a regimen that reduces the strain on your weakened heart and improves your heart's ability to do its work.

For most people, this means following a MAWDS plan every day:

M
Take your MEDICATIONS

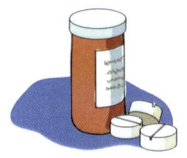

A
Stay ACTIVE each day

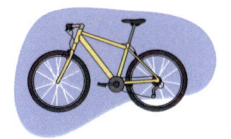

W
WEIGH yourself each day

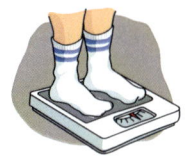

D
Follow your DIET

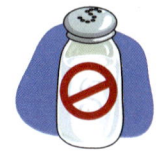

S
Recognize your SYMPTOMS

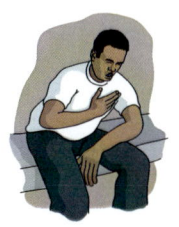

Your medications are proven to help improve your quality and length of life. It's vital that you take your medications exactly as prescribed. Missing a dose, or taking too much, can cause serious problems.

In fact, not taking your medications as instructed is one of the most common reasons people with heart failure need to be hospitalised.

Source: Intermountain Healthcare – Living with Heart Failure

LIFESTYLE MANAGEMENT

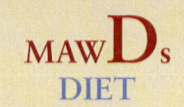

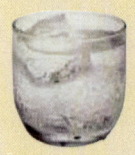

MAWDs DIET

Re-Thinking water drinking

In general, drinking water is good for you. But it's a myth that everyone should drink a lot of water to "flush out the kidneys." And that common prescription to "drink more water" does NOT apply to people with heart failure.

To ease symptoms, people with heart failure need to limit - not increase - the fluids they take in. Use the tips on these pages for what to do when you're thirsty.

1 Limiting your fluid intake

Another way to reduce the fluid retention caused by your heart failure is to drink less fluid – only 8 cups a day (64 ounces). Keep in mind that feeling thirsty doesn't mean your body needs more fluid. So instead of drinking liquids when you're thirsty, try these alternatives:

- Chewing gum
- Sucking on ice chips or hard candy
- Rinsing your mouth with water

The table at the bottom of this page shows an example of how your fluid intake can add up to 64 ounces a day. As you can see, this still allows you to drink a fairly normal amount of fluid per day.

2 Limiting your alcohol consumption

Here are a couple of good reasons to limit your alcohol intake to one drink per day:

- It helps limit your fluid intake to reduce the strain on your heart.
- It prevents heart muscle damage that may be caused by more-than-moderate alcohol use.

Your one-drink limit allows one beer, glass of wine, or cocktail each day. (Note: if alcohol was the cause of your heart failure, stay away from alcohol completely.)

Here's a sample of how fluid intake can add up to your 64-ounce limit:

Breakfast	Lunch	Dinner	Snacks
1 cup = 8 ounces	1 glass water = 12 ounces	1 glass wine = 8 ounces	1 can soda = 12 ounces
1 cup cocoa = 8 ounces	1 cup soup = 8 ounces	1 glass water = 8 ounces	
Subtotal: 16 ounces	Subtotal: 20 ounces	Subtotal: 16 ounces	Subtotal: 12 ounces

Total daily fluids: 64 ounces (1.8 litres)

> **In my own experience, heart failure creates a strange sense of slow motion where the pace of life becomes less frenetic, and we are forced into a more observant and considered state. We so often take for granted the body's ability to move quickly from one position to another, from one speed to another and all whilst being unconscious of these marvels. Then suddenly it dawns on you that these simple acts are now no longer possible, and your only memory is when they had been effortless.**

Sometimes I dream about running only to wake with a rapidly beating heart. I miss the ability to move swiftly and feel free. It's quite hard not to feel vulnerable when you are no longer able to run away. Life takes on new meaning. The hopes and dreams of the past are often abandoned, only to be replaced with surviving from day to day. The speed of modern life, the jostling for position, the misguided perception of food as merely fuel to sustain an over-stressed body, the cosmetic procedures to cling on to the concept of youth, blissfully ignoring its own mortality; all these superficial obsessions pale into insignificance as more authentic issues become important. Of course, if you could predict how long you had left, you might plan your life differently. No one has all the answers.

Despite being given a statistical chance of survival in the US (it seems the Brits are less keen on this openness), a 50% chance of death in 5 years is just that, there's also a 50% chance of surviving too. When right ventricular function is affected it often negatively influences the prognosis considerably. However, I decided early on not to dwell on the statistics but rather to concentrate on optimising my health through the understanding of diet, exercise and mindfulness, as well as the determination to do what I can when I am feeling well (see Chapters 20-26). There are moments of extreme disappointment when a relapse occurs. The first time it happened, I put it down to a simple upper respiratory infection that triggered the exaggerated immune response. However, the second time I had no answers, and this makes it even more difficult to accept.

CHAPTER 20

"Everything in excess is opposed to nature."

Hippocrates

I am dedicating this whole chapter to salt as I got into serious trouble and made my condition far worse through incognisance of the quantities of salt I had been consuming.

It is a well-known fact that sodium is essential to life. It maintains fluid levels and promotes the signalling of nerves throughout the body. That said, the modern diet often contains far too much salt for our needs. There are a few rare occasions when sodium needs to be replenished: e.g., in the cases of severe vomiting and diarrhoea, extreme exercise and overconsumption of water, but only usually on a temporary basis. These cases are relatively rare, and not only is sodium important but the correct balance of electrolytes – magnesium, sodium, potassium, calcium, phosphorus, chloride, and bicarbonate – is essential for good health and the proper functioning of the heart.

So many people have come to the defence of salt in my conversations with them. Here are some of their comments:

- 'But you need salt in your diet'
- 'Not enough salt can cause serious problems too'
- 'I couldn't possibly not add salt to my food it would be tasteless'
- 'I haven't got high blood pressure, so I don't need to worry'
- 'I'm not sick like you – my body can take it'
- 'If I use salt, I only use Himalayan rock salt or sea salt which is much better for you.'

The American Heart Association advises that over 75% of sodium intake is already present in processed and prepared foods and therefore, it is unlikely that anyone would be deficient. Pink Himalayan rock salt and sea salt are both quite fashionable but are chemically very similar to table salt as they still contain up to 98 percent sodium chloride. Consequently, this means that only 2% of these salts are made up of various trace minerals.

I should also mention the plethora of television chefs who add handfuls of salt to any dish at the earliest opportunity even though many of the ingredients used, e.g., capers, olives, pancetta, and parmesan cheese, to name just a few, provide plenty of salt to the dish without needing to add more. You may have also heard that too much sodium is harmful in cases of hypertension. But how much is too much?

The recommended daily allowance (RDA) in the UK is 6g of salt for a healthy adult. In the US the Mayo Clinic recommends 2.5g of sodium for a healthy adult. Herein lies some of the confusion. Sodium and salt are not measured in the same way. Therefore, if a product is listed as sodium, the quantity of sodium needs to be multiplied by 2.4 to obtain the quantity of salt. In the cases of those with high blood pressure, heart failure or kidney problems the recommendation is to consume no more than 0.8g of sodium daily or 2g of salt.

If you've ever wondered why you look and feel swollen the day after eating a salty meal, then look no further than the quantity of salt you may have consumed. As an example, your meal may have begun with some salted crackers, nuts, and olives, followed by cured meats or smoked salmon with capers, followed by an oriental main course with fish and/or soy sauce and end with a salted caramel dessert. You may also have consumed a little alcohol. It is likely that you will spend all night drinking water to alleviate a severely dry mouth and the following day you may have swollen eyelids, look bloated and feel the worse for wear. Sometimes it can be as simple as that. Excess salt can cause havoc on the body's delicate systems as detailed below.

Salt's Effects on the Body

ARTERIES

The extra blood pressure caused by eating too much salt puts extra strain on the inside of your arteries. To cope with the extra strain, the tiny muscles in the artery walls become stronger and thicker. Yet this only makes the space inside the arteries smaller and raises your blood pressure even higher. This cycle of increasing blood pressure (which occurs slowly over a number of years) can ultimately lead to the arteries bursting or becoming so narrow that they can clog up entirely. When this happens, the organs of the body that were receiving the blood from the arteries become starved of the oxygen and nutrients they need. This can result in the organs being damaged and can be fatal.

Source: Blood Pressure UK

KIDNEYS

Salt's Effects on the Body

Your body removes unwanted fluid by filtering your blood through your kidneys. Here any extra fluid is sucked out and put into your bladder to be removed as urine.

To do this, your kidneys use osmosis to draw the extra water out of your blood. This process uses a delicate balance of sodium and potassium to pull the water across a wall of cells from the bloodstream into a collecting channel that leads to the bladder.

Eating salt raises the amount of sodium in your bloodstream and wrecks the delicate balance, reducing the ability of your kidneys to remove the water.

The result is a higher blood pressure due to the extra fluid and extra strain on the delicate blood vessels leading to the kidneys. Over time, this extra strain can damage the kidneys – known as kidney disease. This reduces their ability to filter out unwanted and toxic waste products, which then start to build up in the body.

If kidney disease is left untreated and the blood pressure isn't lowered, the damage can lead to kidney failure. This is when the kidneys are no longer able to filter the blood and the body slowly becomes poisoned by its own toxic waste products. If you have high blood pressure and are being treated with a diuretic medication, this makes the kidneys remove more fluid from the bloodstream. Because the sodium in salt counteracts this effect, reducing your salt intake will make your blood pressure medicine more effective.

Source: Blood Pressure UK

Salt's Effects on the Body

HEART

The raised blood pressure caused by eating too much salt may damage the arteries leading to the heart.

At first, it may cause a slight reduction in the amount of blood reaching the heart. This may lead to angina (sharp pains in the chest when being active).

With this condition the cells in the heart don't work as well as they should because they are not receiving enough oxygen and nutrients. However, lowering blood pressure may help to alleviate some of the problems and reduce the risk of greater damage.

If you continue to eat too much salt then, over time, the damage caused by the extra blood pressure may become so severe that the arteries burst or become completely clogged.

If this happens, then the part of the heart that was receiving the blood no longer gets the oxygen and nutrients it needs and dies. The result is a heart attack.

The best way to prevent a heart attack is to stop the arteries becoming damaged. And one of the best ways of doing this is to keep your blood pressure down by eating less salt.

Source: Blood Pressure UK

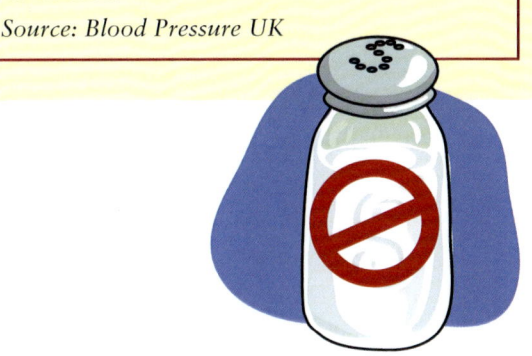

Salt's Effects on the Body

BRAIN

The raised blood pressure caused by eating too much salt may damage the arteries leading to the brain.

At first, it may cause a slight reduction in the amount of blood reaching the brain. This may lead to dementia (known as vascular dementia).

With this condition the cells in the brain don't work as well as they should because they are not receiving enough oxygen and nutrients. However, lowering blood pressure may help to alleviate some of the problems and reduce the risk of greater damage.

If you continue to eat too much salt then, over time, the damage caused by the extra blood pressure may become so severe that the arteries burst or become completely clogged.

If this happens, then the part of the brain that was receiving the blood no longer gets the oxygen and nutrients it needs and dies. The result is a stroke, where you lose the ability to do the things that part of the brain used to control.

The best way to prevent a stroke is to stop the arteries becoming damaged. And one of the best ways of doing this is keep your blood pressure down by eating less salt.

Source: Blood Pressure UK

So how do you eat a low-salt diet?

I would agree that it is rather difficult. There is an inordinate amount of salt in so many of the foods we consume daily. We live in a society where salt-laden, ready-prepared meals have become commonplace. Thanks to modern labelling we can actively monitor our own individual salt intake, but even the labels can be confusing to someone inexperienced in reading them and that's why I often use a calculator at the supermarket.

After only a short period, taste buds adjust to less salt, and it becomes easier to learn which foods to avoid. That doesn't mean missing out on all the foods we love. For example, I am very fond of crab, but the average portion of crab (100grams) contains approximately one gram of salt. Therefore, if I eat crab on one day, I make sure all my other meals throughout the day are low in salt so that it doesn't cause a problem. However, there are foods which are notoriously high in salt and in my opinion questionable as to their nutritional value. Here is a list of the foods I no longer eat or in very small quantities:

- **Bacon and cured meats** – on average bacon contains approximately one gram of salt per rasher and cured raw ham contains up to 12 grams of salt per serving.
- **Fish sauce and soy sauce** – it's mind-boggling how much salt they contain! As an alternative I sometimes use low-salt gluten free soy sauce and just a teaspoon will go a long way in enhancing flavour. Alternatively, adding a good quality balsamic vinegar will work well in some dishes.

- **Smoked salmon and caviar** – alas two things I love which are very high in salt – now I eat just a mouthful of smoked salmon very occasionally.
- **Stock cubes** – I make my own stock and use garlic, onions, and shallots for flavour.
- **Bread** – unless you make your own bread and know how much salt it contains. Even if you can read the label, two slices of bread may contain 1g of salt, adding a large amount to your daily salt intake without your realising it.
- **Cheese** – the only cheeses I now eat in very small quantities are grated parmesan, mozzarella, and mascarpone. As parmesan is often used grated, a little goes a long way and a teaspoon added to a dish can make all the difference in imparting its umami flavour. I don't always recommend the ready grated variety as it sometimes smells like old socks and has very little flavour. Buy the best parmesan you can afford, keep it sealed in the fridge and grate a little as desired.
- **Pickles and olives** – there are a couple of Californian companies who produce low-sodium olives. I buy capers in vinegar and rinse copiously to remove excess salt before using them in very small amounts.
- **Sodas and soft drinks** may contain a lot of salt as well as some OTC medications, e.g., soluble acetaminophen and antacids. Always check the labels.
- **Soup** – I don't know why but most of the soups available to buy are laden with salt. The safest way to eat soup is to make your own – see pages 221 and 223 for suggestions.

Breakfast...

Researchers at Harvard University say that missing breakfast may put an 'extra strain' on the heart, sending it into a protective drive that raises blood pressure, insulin levels and cholesterol – all of which can lead to heart disease.

I have singled out breakfast as I have found it quite difficult to eat a low salt breakfast, especially when away from home. So many of the modern breakfast cereals are packed with salt, even though they may be advertised as having various health benefits. Having to avoid gluten also makes it twice as difficult.

Likewise, the traditional English and American breakfast often contains too much salt. For example, two sausages, two rashers of bacon, scrambled eggs, brown sauce, toast/English muffin equate to at least four and a half grams of salt. By adding a portion of baked beans, this takes it up to around seven grams of salt. Considering that six grams is the maximum daily allowance for healthy people, this quantity of salt would be totally inappropriate for those with a heart condition, who should eat no more than 2 grams daily. By the end of the day, the total salt consumed would be enormous and oedema would result as the heart struggles to cope with all the excess fluid.

It is relatively easy to find a healthy lunch or dinner when away from home, for example fish/meat and steamed vegetables, but as breakfast is more problematic, I have provided some examples of healthy breakfasts overleaf which might inspire you.

Breakfast Suggestions
- Baked mackerel (rich in omega-3)
- Poached eggs with spinach, drizzled with olive oil
- Mixed berries with kefir and pistachio/macadamia nuts
- Scrambled eggs with mushrooms and grilled tomatoes
- Miles River omelette (see recipe page 219)

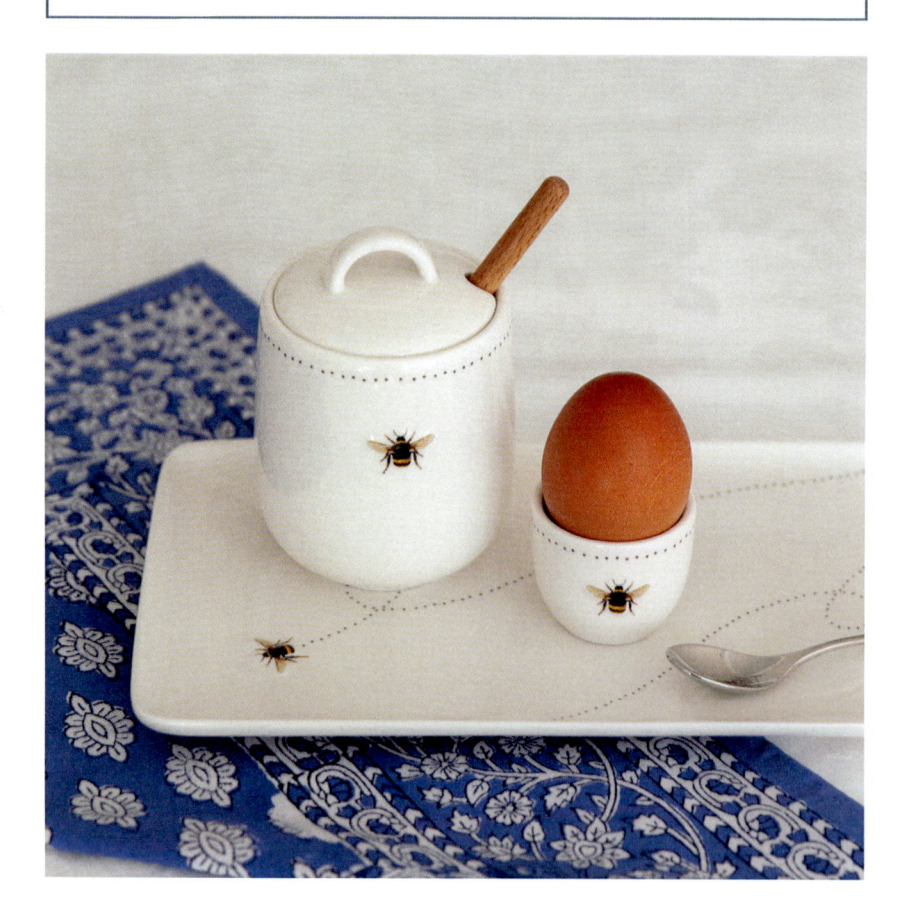

CHAPTER 21

"Let food be thy medicine and medicine be thy food."

Hippocrates

The earth has provided us with an abundance of wonderful food which is designed to sustain and nourish our bodies. Unfortunately, in the last 50 years the food industry has often experimented with our food and has sometimes changed the molecular structure to such an extent that some processed foods have become particularly harmful whilst purporting to be healthy, e.g., margarine. The incidence of heart disease, obesity, diabetes and autoimmune illnesses has grown in direct correlation to the changes in our diets. It is quite sad to think that we may have been misled and encouraged to eat products that have been quite harmful to our health e.g., trans fats, excess sugar, excess salt, pesticide-laden fruits and vegetables, microplastic contaminated water and fish, fruit juices, sodas, factory oils and much more. The way food is grown also has a significant impact on quality and nutritional value.

Moreover, scientists do not always agree what is healthy and what is not. There is often individual variability which makes deciphering the science even more difficult with so many conflicting theories. Many books have been written about how food affects your body, from leaky gut, to lectins, to complex carbohydrates, to high protein, low protein, vegan, gluten, sugar, salt, fasting, low carbohydrate, etc. The list is endless, and no one has all the answers. Considering all the conflicting information we face daily, it might be easy to develop orthorexia nervosa, an eating disorder characterised by an excessive preoccupation with eating healthy food.

Let's take the example of the humble tomato: If you are following a lectin-free diet, removing the seeds and skin would enable you to enjoy the flesh and obtain the health benefits. However, tomatoes are also members of the nightshade family and may cause inflammation in some individuals. Of course, we have all now been told that whole tomatoes are extremely good for us as they have a high lycopene content, a red pigment of the carotene class of compounds which may be protective against heart and eye disease, and some cancers. This is just one example of how confusing the information we receive might be. Furthermore, when you are navigating a serious illness, it is essential to eat a diet that will not exacerbate your condition and help you onto the road to recover. As I mentioned in Chapter 10, I worsened my heart failure by eating too much salt during a three-week stay in Cyprus, without even realising it.

After my own personal research, I have discovered that 'leaky gut' and chronic inflammation may play a significant role in a variety of autoimmune illnesses. Leaky gut allows endotoxins (e.g., lipopolysaccharides) to pass across the gut barrier into the blood stream and play havoc with the immune system. However, this theory is still considered to be outside of the mainstream although many functional doctors seem to concur. The other problem is that many medical doctors, even to this day, receive very little education on nutrition while studying medicine, despite the obvious importance to health and well-being. As of 2020, I have been heartened to learn that first- and second-year medical students at the University of Maryland School of Medicine (UMSOM) have a new requirement to earn their medical degree – culinary medicine. It's certainly a step in the right direction and I hope other universities will emphasise the importance of nutrition in their curricula also.

Moreover, we are still learning such a lot about the immune system, and from the Covid-19 experience, I am hoping that scientists will discover much more about how the immune system works and how it starts attacking itself.

The effects of chemicals in our environment, e.g., pesticides and estrogen-mimicking compounds may either suppress or inappropriately stimulate the immune system, both of which may be dangerous to those with autoimmune disease. Furthermore, GM foods (e.g., wheat which has been genetically modified to grow shorter in height and in turn produce more gluten) and environmental chemicals may have all played a role in making us more sensitive to the foods that we eat.

Research is ongoing and we continue to learn and understand the importance of provenance and environmental impacts on the food we consume. However, it is very difficult to navigate when one study says, for example, that eggs are healthy one week and unhealthy the next.

So, what do you eat?

I am a great believer in everything in moderation. Likewise, you should observe which foods appear to exacerbate your condition and learn how to avoid them.

Although I enjoyed baking cakes while I was growing up, I learnt how to cook savoury meals in Provence while I was studying French. I had the good fortune to spend my sojourn with an authentic Mediterranean family and the grandmother, Mémé Simone, would often come to stay and share her wonderful recipes with me.

There is something truly generous about sharing food. It's the one thing which cuts through boundaries, brings people together and with the combined efforts of those involved often provides a sense of achievement and fulfilment, not to mention satisfying one's appetite.

It's a pity our modern lifestyle is eclipsing these traditions. Those who don't know how to cook are at a huge disadvantage when it comes to optimising one's health, despite the plethora of wonderful cookery books available with easy-to-follow recipes. Many foods possess powerful healing qualities, e.g., sour cherries for gout, cranberries for urinary tract infections, beetroot to help dilate the blood vessels and the powerful anti-inflammatory effects of garlic, turmeric, and ginger to name just a few. However, whilst these foods may have a positive effect for certain conditions, in some cases their power may have a negative effect on others. Cherries may upset some with gastrointestinal issues due to their sorbitol content, grapefruit and cranberries are contraindicated when taken with certain medications and garlic may not be suitable for those following a FODMAP diet or whilst on anticoagulants. It's a minefield out there, there is so much to consider.

While researching food that might help my health, I have discovered many wonderful cookery books and have made a note of some of the ones I found particularly helpful on pages 273 and 274. However, although I am neither a trained nutritionist nor a famous chef, I have learnt a lot about the benefits of certain foods and enjoy cooking and inventing recipes. Therefore, I would like to share with you several of my favourite recipes; some are invented, some adapted, some provided by friends, and some have been kindly given to me during my travels. The emphasis in all the recipes is that they are low in salt and carbohydrate and free from gluten. They are easy to follow and finally, despite the absence of salt, according to Joaquin they still taste delicious (except my risotto, a recipe I have not included ☺). I do hope you have fun making them.

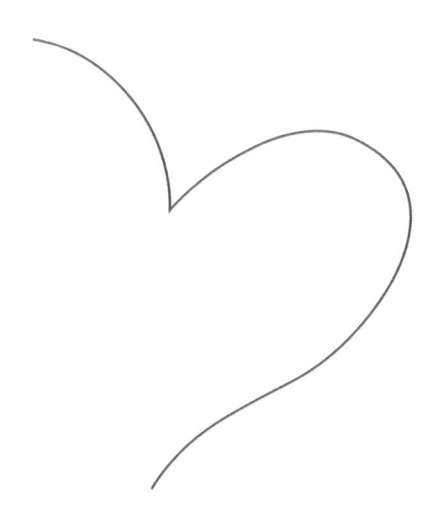

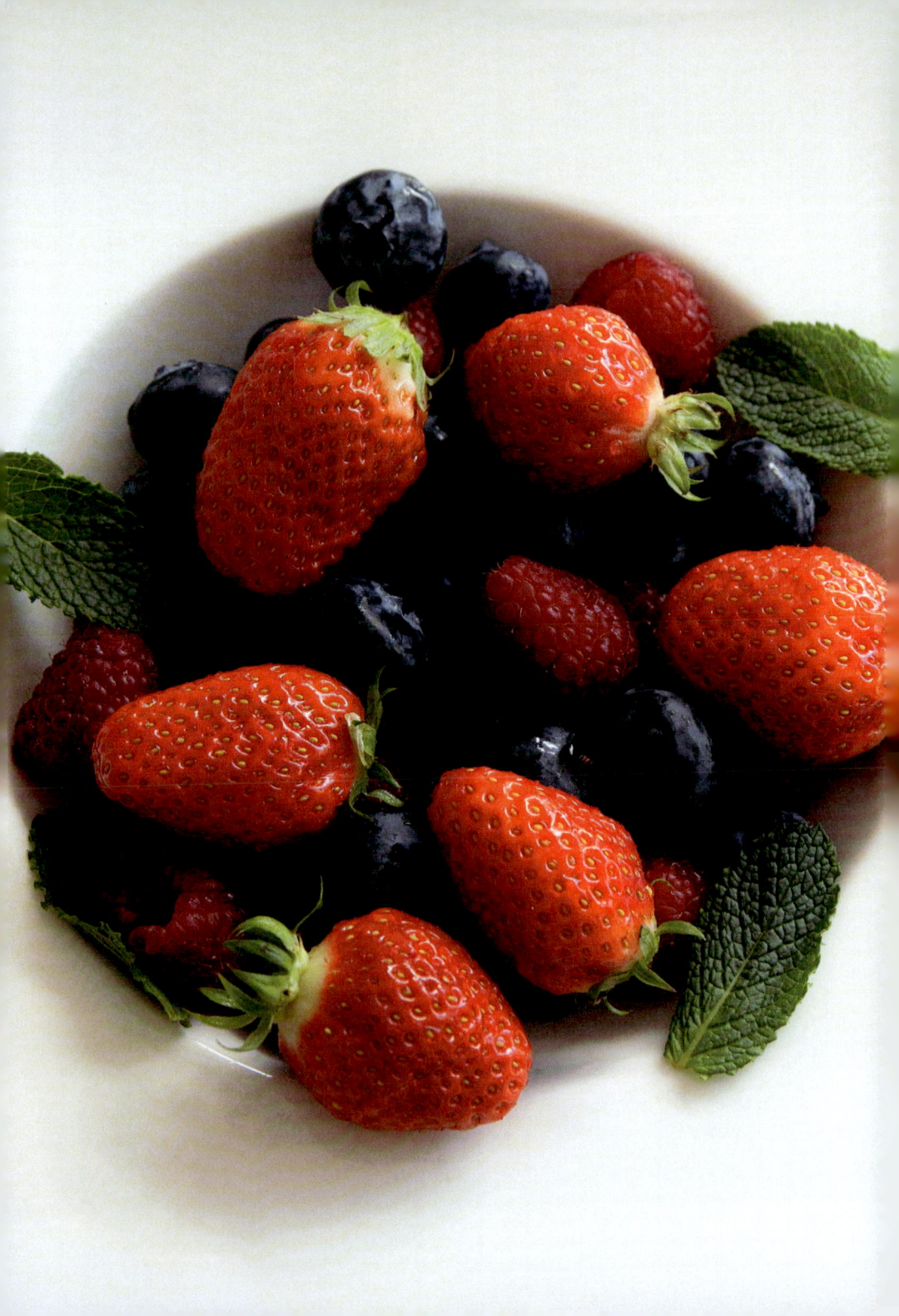

Happy Heart Recipes

Miles River Omelette
219

Waterfall Watercress Soup
221

Vegetable Soup
223

Seafood Brochettes
225

Oriental Shrimp
226

Salmon Curry with Papaya and Lime
228

Roast Lamb with Rosemary
231

Salsa Verde and Chimichurri Sauces
232/233

Blueberry and Almond Cake
235

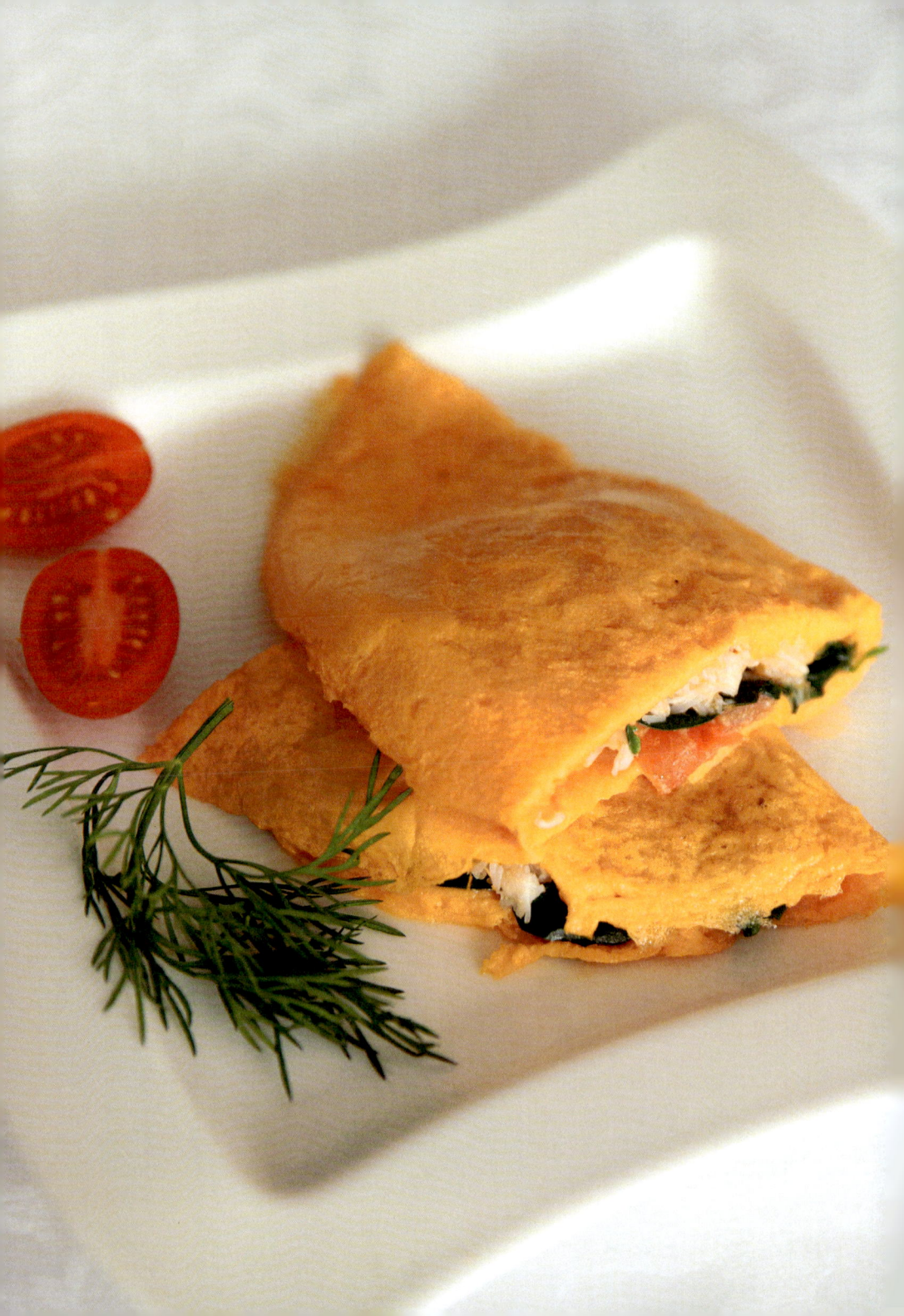

Miles River Omelette

2 eggs
1 teaspoon of unsalted butter
1 portion of lightly steamed spinach
1 tomato skinned, deseeded, and cubed
30 grams of fresh white crabmeat
freshly ground black pepper

Serves 1

Steam the spinach and cubed tomato to warm through for approx. 3 minutes. Set aside and keep warm.

Lightly beat the eggs together in a small bowl. Melt the butter in an omelette pan over a medium heat. Pour in the beaten eggs and cook without stirring until the omelette starts to bubble around the edges, about 30 seconds. Then gather the mixture towards the centre of the pan and allow the uncooked part to cover the pan again, making sure to keep the omelette in one piece. This should take about one to two minutes. When the bottom has set but the top is still slightly wet, place the spinach, tomato, and crab mixture on one side of the omelette and then fold over the other half of the omelette to cover the filling. Cook until the filling is heated through. Slide the omelette onto a plate, season with pepper, and serve immediately.

Chef's Note:

I ate something similar to this recipe while staying in the Chesapeake Bay area of Maryland, where crabs are large, plentiful, and delicious.

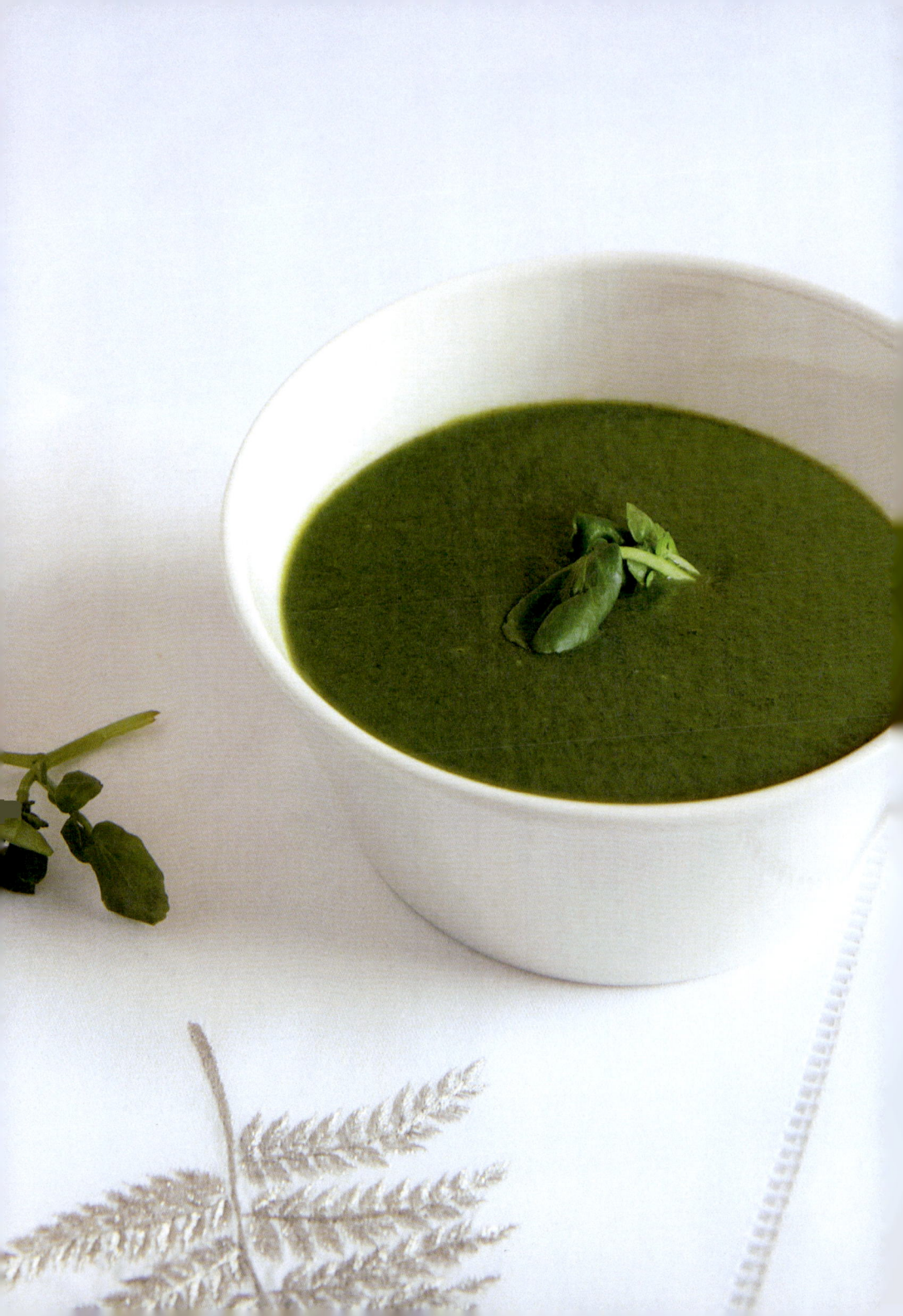

Waterfall Watercress Soup

1 chopped red onion
2 small potatoes, peeled
(cooked rice may be substituted)
500ml of chicken or vegetable stock
200 grams of good quality watercress
woody stalks removed
1 tablespoon of olive oil
freshly ground black pepper

Serves 2–3

Boil the potatoes in a small pan until tender, drain and set aside. Heat the oil in a large frying pan on a medium heat. Add the onion and cook until soft, then add the stock and bring to the boil. Add the cooked potatoes and bring back to the boil. Remove from the heat, add the watercress immediately, cover with a lid and leave for 5–7 minutes until the watercress has wilted. This step will help retain the vitamins and vibrant green colour. Pour the mixture, after it has cooled a little, into a liquidiser and blend until smooth. Reheat gently and serve immediately with freshly ground black pepper.

Chef's Note:

This must be the quickest and easiest soup recipe I have ever made. It is excellent for removing excess fluid from the body, if required, and has numerous health benefits including being rich in iron, minerals, and vitamin K.

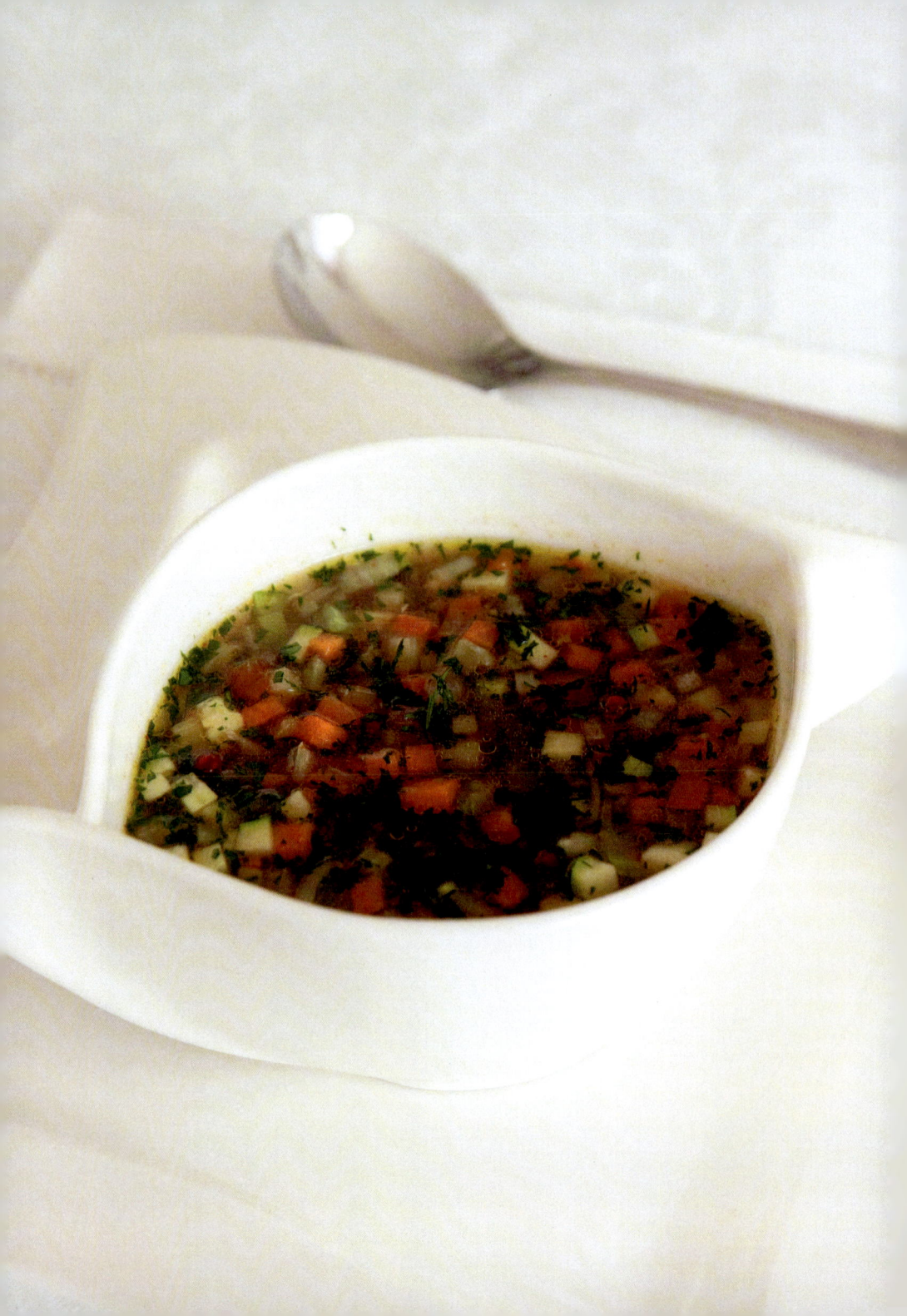

Vegetable Soup

500ml of stock – vegetable, beef or chicken
sofrito: 1 onion, 6 carrots and 3 celery stalks chopped into small cubes
2 tablespoons of olive oil
3 medium tomatoes, skinned, deseeded, and cubed
1 fresh chilli pepper
2 tablespoons of tomato purée
2 waxy potatoes, cubed
1 courgette, cubed
1 teaspoon of ground cumin
1–2 garlic cloves, peeled and finely chopped
1 teaspoon of pink peppercorns
Parsley and dill, finely chopped

Serves 3

Fry the sofrito in a pan with 2 tablespoons of olive oil. Adjust the oil as required. When the sofrito has softened slightly, stir in the garlic, tomato and cumin. Heat through without burning. Add the stock and bring to the boil. Turn down to simmer, add the chilli pepper, tomato purée, peppercorns, and potatoes. Cook for approx. 15 minutes. Add the courgette and parsley and simmer until tender. Sprinkle with freshly chopped dill prior to serving.

Chef's Note:

This is a very versatile soup. It may be eaten on its own, with a sprinkling of parmesan or used as a base in which to poach salmon or other seafood to make a wholesome meal. Other vegetables may be added, e.g. Romanesco, cauliflower, cavolo nero, asparagus, peas, etc, depending on what you might have available in your refrigerator.

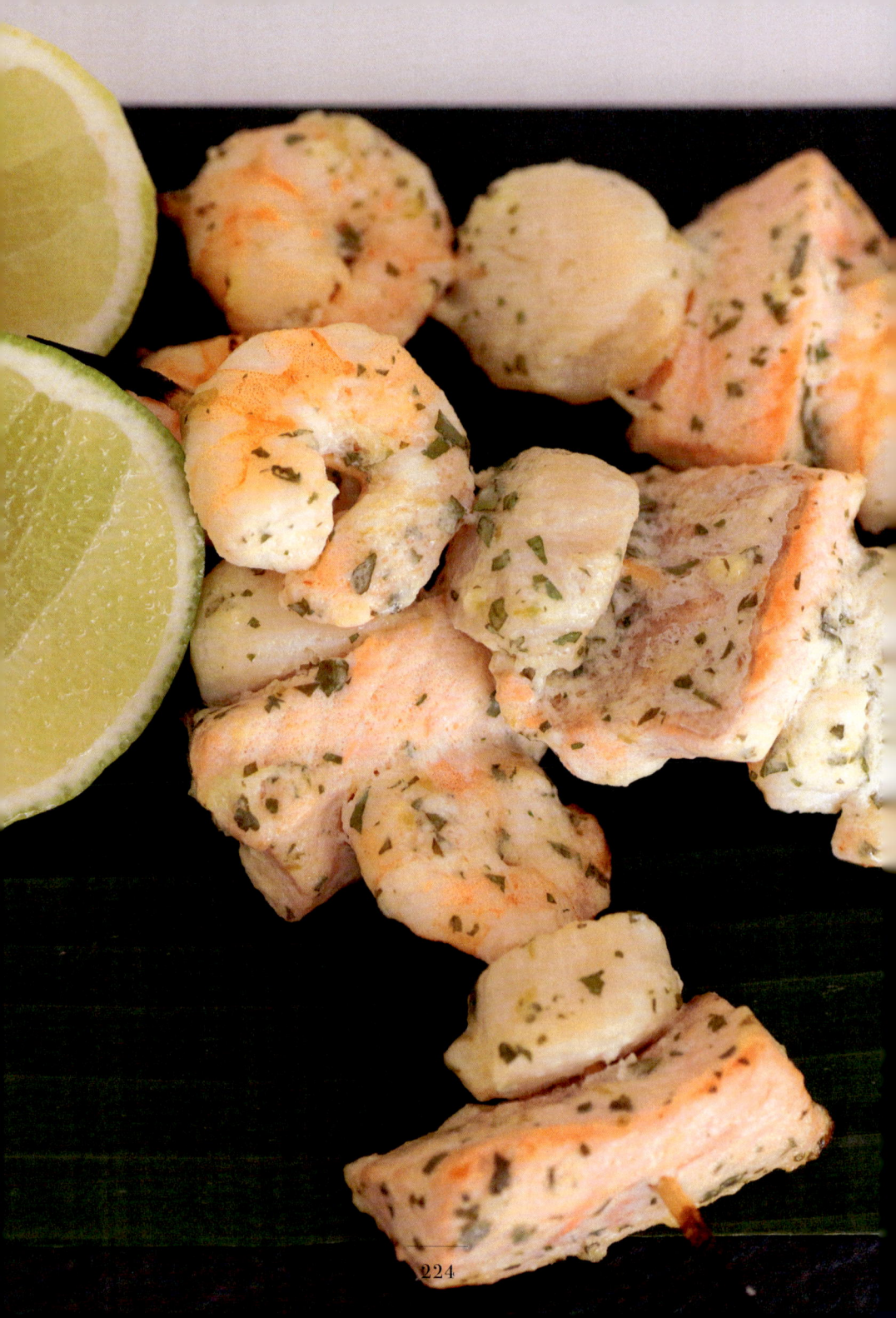

Seafood Brochettes

Assorted seafood of your choice: scallops, shrimp, and monkfish, as a suggestion, to make eight skewers.

Serves 4

Marinade:
½ glass white wine
1 cup yoghurt
2 cloves garlic (3–4 if small)
½ bunch coriander
1 teaspoon arrowroot (to thicken)
1 lump fresh ginger (approx. 2 x size of garlic)
2 tablespoons of olive oil
zest of 1 lime

Chop, crush, and blend marinade ingredients together. Thread seafood onto thin bamboo skewers. Marinade the skewers in mixture for 2–6 hours (optional). Preheat the oven to 200°C (425°F). Place the skewers on a baking tray lined with foil and bake for 10–15 minutes, turning over the skewers mid-way. Finish off under a high grill for 2–3 minutes, to brown them.

Chef's Note:

This recipe was given to me by my friend Geoff in Washington, DC. It's perfect as a delicious starter or light supper.

Oriental Shrimp

1 teaspoon of Sichuan peppercorns
4 spring onions (scallions)
4 dried whole Sichuan chillies (6/10 heat), cut into pieces
1 chunk of ginger, chopped finely
2 garlic cloves, chopped finely
2 tablespoons of olive oil
8 medium-sized asparagus
150g of raw, peeled, and deveined king prawns (or shrimp)
Thai, basmati, or cauliflower rice (quantity according to preference)
1 tablespoon of chopped roasted hazelnuts
1 lime, zest, and juice
1 teaspoon of cornflour (corn starch)
2 tablespoons of water
1 teaspoon of caster sugar
1 tablespoon of rice vinegar (salt-free version)
1 teaspoon of gluten-free, low-salt tamari soy sauce

Serves 2

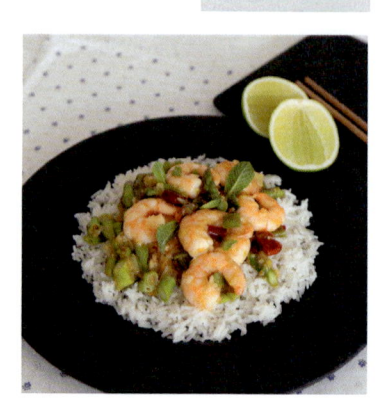

Wash the spring onions and chop into 1cm pieces. Separate the white part from the dark green and set aside. Chop the Sichuan chillies, ginger and garlic and add to the white part of the spring onions. Rinse the raw prawns thoroughly to remove the excess salt and pat dry. Clean and chop the asparagus into 1-inch pieces. Place the roasted hazelnuts into a bowl with the dark green part of the spring onions.

Prepare the sauce by firstly combining the cornflour and water together in a bowl, taking care to blend any lumps, then add the sugar and mix well. Finally add the vinegar and soy sauce. The amount of salt in the recipe will be dictated by the quantity and quality of soy sauce.

Prepare and cook the rice. Blanch the asparagus for 1 minute in a pan of boiling water, cool them rapidly with cold water, drain and set aside. It is important to prepare all items in advance and have them close to the pan as the cooking stage goes very quickly.

Heat the oil in a large wok on a medium to high heat and add the Sichuan peppercorns to flavour the oil. This should take approx. 2–3 minutes. Discard the peppercorns but retain the oil. On a medium heat, add the Sichuan chillies, ginger, garlic, and white part of the spring onions to the oil in the pan and cook for 3–4 minutes; stir regularly taking care not to burn the garlic. Add the prawns and make sure they are cooked on both sides (they will turn pink and no longer look transparent). Stir the sauce briskly and add to the pan. Heat through while stirring until piping hot. Add the asparagus, green part of the spring onions, lime zest and roasted hazelnuts, heat through and serve in bowls with the rice and a liberal squeeze of fresh lime.

Chef's Note:

Chicken/beef/pork may be substituted for prawns but should be cooked separately before adding to the dish just prior to the sauce. One of the challenges of a low-salt diet is eating oriental food. Whilst every effort has been made to reduce the salt in this recipe, the salt content is still moderate, and therefore it would probably be wise to eat this dish as a special treat.

Salmon Curry with Papaya and Lime

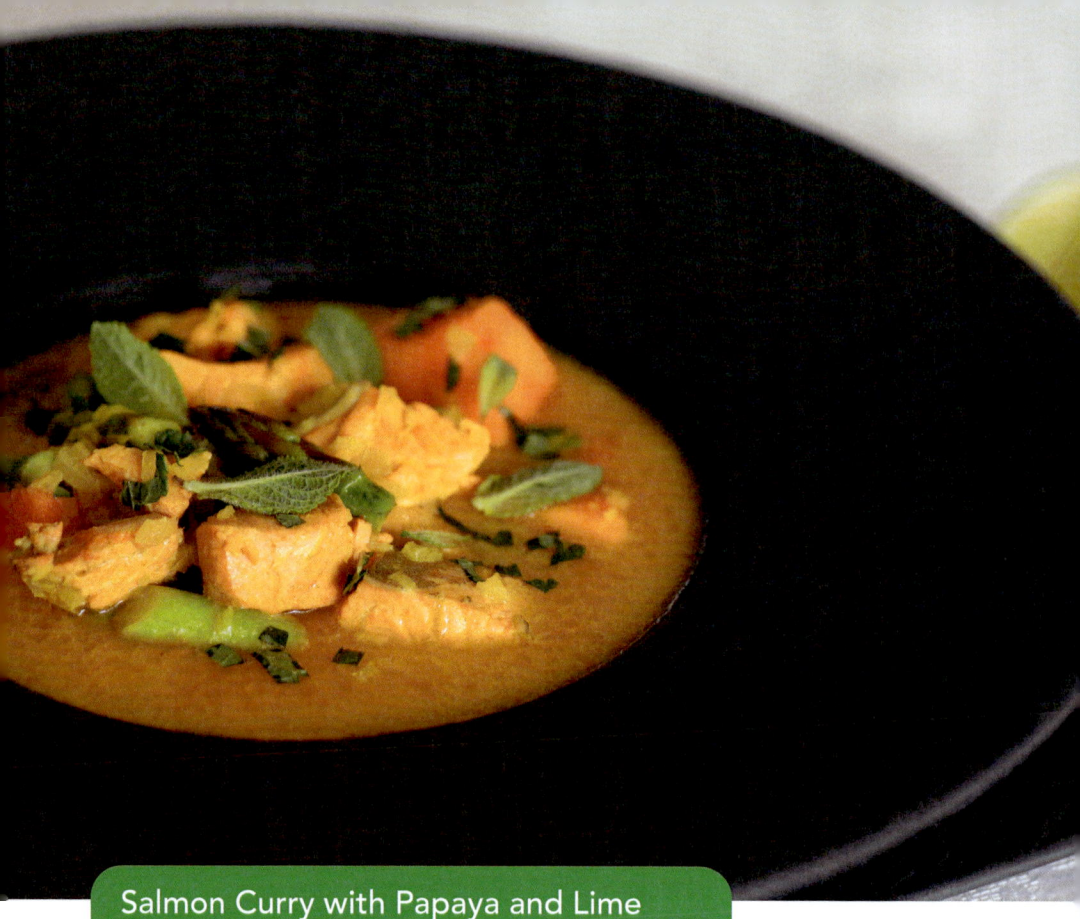

Serves 4

450g (1 lb) fillet of salmon
2 tablespoons olive oil
1 garlic clove, finely chopped (green shoot removed)
1 medium/large onion, skinned and finely chopped
2 tablespoons fresh ginger, finely chopped
1 teaspoon chopped lemongrass (tender root only)
1 whole lemongrass cut into two pieces lengthways
1 teaspoon mild chilli powder
1 teaspoon ground coriander
1 teaspoon ground turmeric
grated zest and juice of 1 lime

400ml (14 fl oz) can of coconut milk (reduced fat coconut milk works well also)
½ ripe papaya, skinned, de-seeded and cut into chunks (no fibrous texture should remain)
8 medium-sized asparagus, chopped into small pieces
2 teaspoons chopped mint

Remove the salmon skin and cut the fish into 2.5cm (1 inch) cubes. Set aside. Heat the oil in a wok or roomy frying pan and add the chopped garlic, onion, and ginger. Let everything fry gently until the ingredients are soft but not brown. Stir together the lemongrass, spices, lime zest and juice and add to the pan. Mix the pan ingredients together over a gentle heat for approx. 1 minute. Add the coconut milk and turn up the heat to bubble up, then turn down the heat and simmer for five minutes. At this point the sauce may be used immediately or set aside (refrigerate if not using immediately). When you are ready to serve, reheat the sauce and add the cubed fish and asparagus. Cover and let it simmer until the fish turns opaque (two to three minutes). Add the papaya to warm through. Sprinkle with chopped mint and serve.

Chef's Note:

This curry is full of anti-inflammatory ingredients and is an excellent dish for a dinner party. It may be served with spiralised courgettes/zucchini or basmati/cauliflower rice

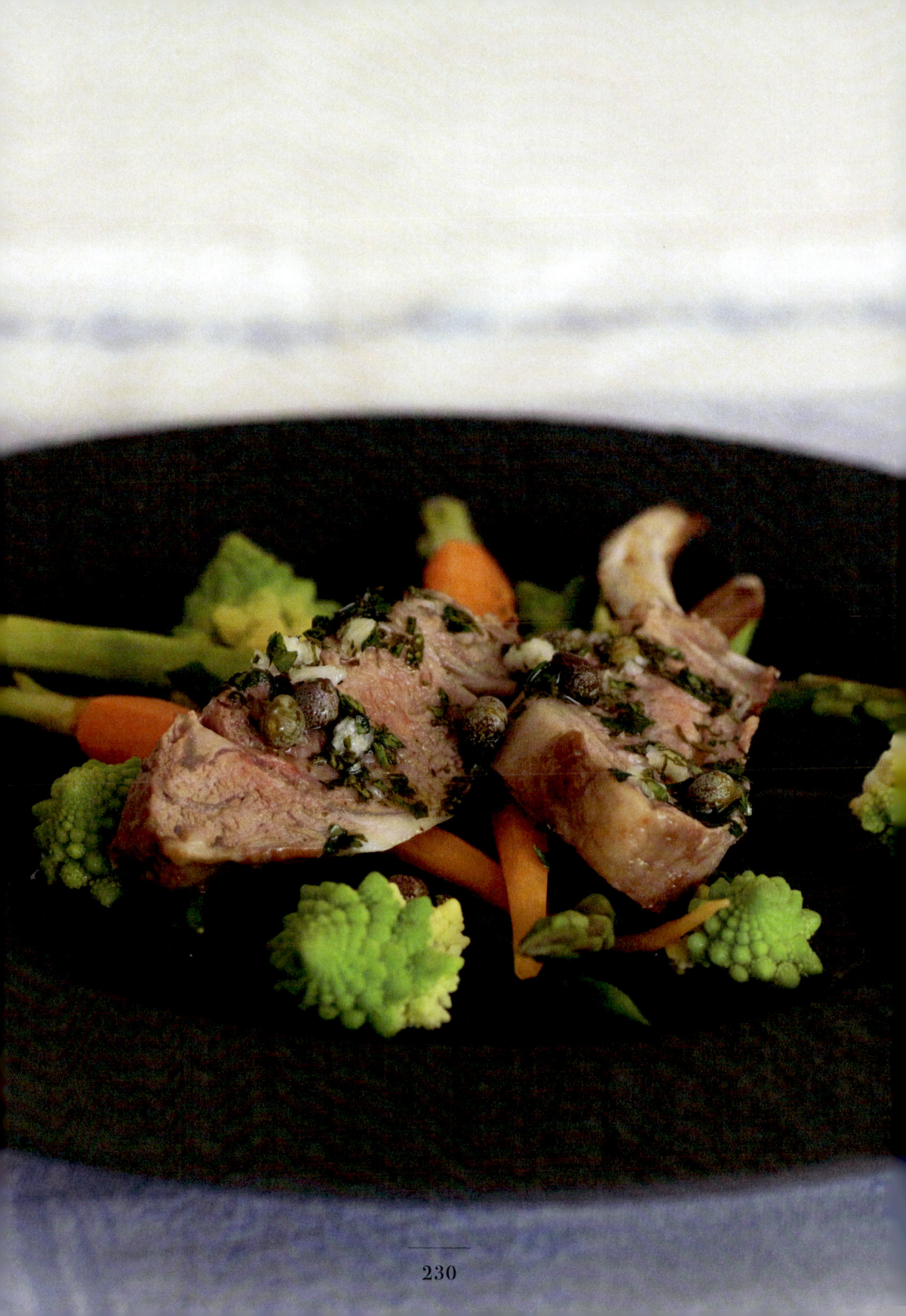

Roast Lamb with Rosemary and Salsa Verde

1 large rack of lamb
rosemary cut into sprigs
2 garlic cloves cut into thin slivers
medley of steamed vegetables, according to preference
salsa verde sauce (see recipe page 232)

Serves 2

Preheat the oven to 200°C (425°F). Place the lamb in a roasting tin, make several openings in the flesh with a pointed knife and insert fine slivers of garlic and sprigs of rosemary, making sure the garlic is below the surface so that it doesn't burn. Drizzle with olive oil and roast the lamb for about 15 minutes for medium rare or longer depending on the size of the rack and your preference. Cover with foil and leave to rest in a warm place for about 10 minutes.

Prepare the salsa verde as per the recipe overleaf. Steam the vegetables and when cooked, set aside and keep warm.

Serve the lamb with the freshly steamed vegetables and a copious serving of the salsa verde sauce. Delicious!

Chef's Note:

This is one of Joaquin's favourites. It's surprisingly easy to make and the salsa verde complements the lamb very well.

Salsa Verde

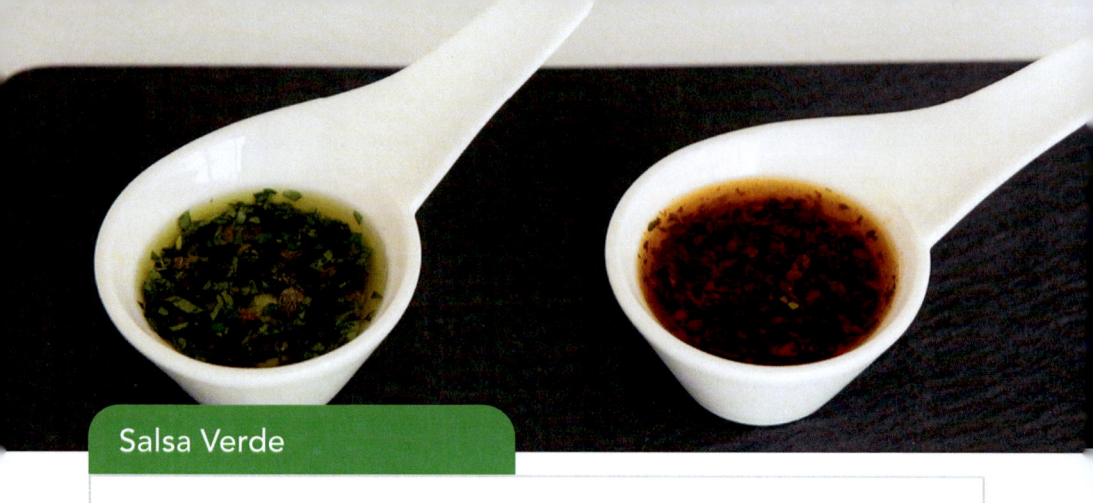

5 tablespoons fruity olive oil
Juice of 1 lemon (approx. 3 tbsp.)
½ teaspoon caster sugar
1 clove garlic, green shoot removed and then crushed
1 tablespoon capers in vinegar (drained and rinsed – see Chef's Note below)
25g (1 oz) flat-leaf parsley, chopped with stalks removed

Pour the lemon juice into a bowl, add the sugar, and stir until dissolved.

Add the olive oil, garlic, capers, and parsley. Set aside at room temperature to infuse. Drizzle over fish or meat as desired.

Chef's Note:

This sauce is a versatile and delicious accompaniment to a wide variety of dishes. It may be served with any fish and is a perfect complement to lamb and pork. Capers are a little salty and I always soak them in boiling water for 5 minutes (and then rinse with cold, to remove the excess salt) before adding to the sauce.
NB: this does not affect the potency of the capers' flavour.

Chimichurri

1 tablespoon of fresh parsley, finely chopped
1 tablespoon of oregano, finely chopped
1 fresh jalapeno chilli, finely chopped
3 tablespoons of red wine vinegar
1 clove garlic, finely grated
1 teaspoon of paprika (adjust according to heat preference)
4 tablespoons of extra virgin olive oil

Place all the ingredients into a bowl without the oil. Mix well and then add the oil and mix until everything floats. Before using, leave the sauce to infuse for at least two hours or overnight. Dry herbs may be substituted if fresh are not available, but the quantities should be adjusted to 1 teaspoon each and a teaspoon of water should be added to the dry ingredients before adding to the mixture.

Chef's Note:

In Argentina chimichurri is typically served with grilled steaks and other meats served at an *asado*. There are many stories about the origin of the word 'chimichurri' such as it being named after 'Jimmy Curry' an Englishman who joined the fight for Argentine Independence, or from the English speaking in 'Spanglish' and asking for curry 'Che mi curry'. Food historians believe that chimichurri using dry herbs was invented by gauchos to flavour meat cooked over open fires. The above recipe was provided by Pablo who makes delicious *asados* at *el campo*.

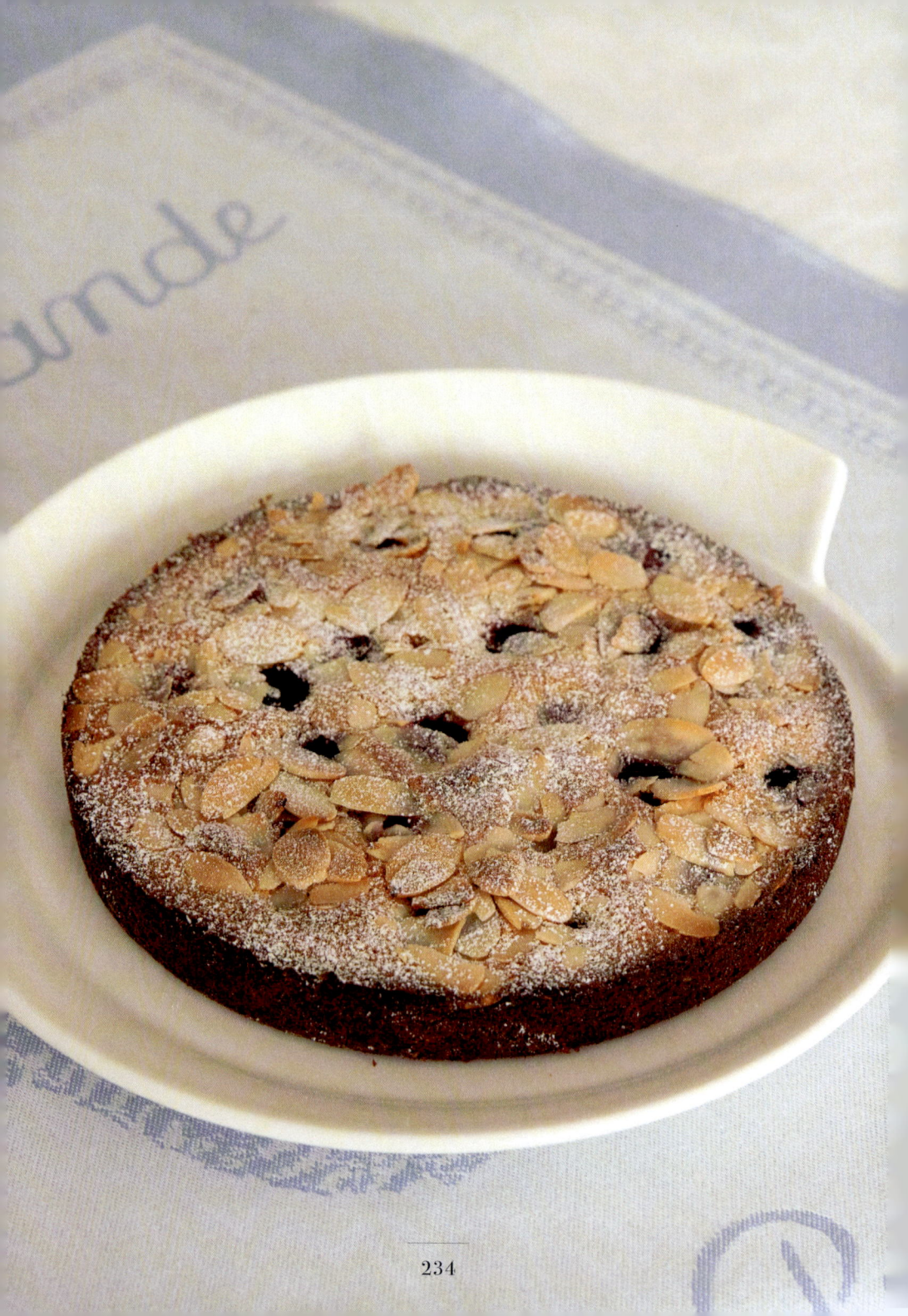

Blueberry and Almond Cake

60 grams of fresh blueberries
75 grams of caster sugar
100 grams of unsalted butter
1 large egg
100 grams of ground almonds
1 teaspoon of cornflour
1 teaspoon of vanilla essence
flaked almonds
icing sugar sieved

Serves 4

Preheat the oven to 190°C (375°F) and place a baking tray on the top shelf to heat through. Line and grease with parchment paper an 18cm/7-inch cake tin with removable bottom and sides and set aside. In a large bowl beat the butter and sugar until smooth, add the egg and mix well, then incorporate the vanilla essence. Mix the ground almonds with the cornflour and then fold into the wet mixture. Spoon the mixture into the cake tin, smooth the top, press the blueberries into the cake mix and sprinkle with ground almonds. Place the tin onto the pre-heated baking tray and bake for approximately 25–30 minutes until golden. Allow to cool before removing carefully from the tin and dust with icing sugar before serving.

Chef's Note:

This cake is naturally gluten-free, easy to make and is simply delicious.

CHAPTER 22

"A kind word to one in trouble is often like a switch in a railroad track... An inch between wreck and smooth sailing."

Henry Ward Beecher

Everyone is unique and when facing a chronic or life-threatening illness, each person may deal with their situation in their own individual way. They may feel a vast array of emotions including shock, disbelief, sorrow, depression, despair, helplessness, isolation, and even guilt. Friends and family usually wish to help but often don't know how to handle you or your new situation. I've experienced this a lot and have written below a list of suggestions which may give some insight to those who are struggling.

The first thing that most people say is 'If there's anything I can do to help, please let me know'. Of course, this is a polite expression and makes the person saying it feel better. However, this invariably leaves the proverbial ball in the sick person's court, and you're unlikely to ring anyone to say 'could you come and make my bed, pick up some groceries, help me do a load of washing or vacuum the carpet,' particularly at the beginning of the illness when you are only just coming to terms with the fact that many of the things you did before with ease now leave you exhausted. I've become a little better at asking people to help and have a few photos of friends who have vacuumed my carpet while I cooked them supper. It's a learning curve. Of course, there are those who offer help but don't mean it and perhaps the only time you ask for their help, they provide a litany of excuses, and you no longer feel confident to ask again. If you are sincere about offering help, in addition to the ideas above, I have made a list below of some of my suggestions:

- **Accompanying your friend/relative on hospital visits. You would need to gauge if this were something they would like/appreciate. Do make sure you are able to allow enough time to do this as there's nothing worse than being abandoned mid-appointment.**

- **Certain household chores can be quite challenging for heart failure patients. Vacuuming, changing/making beds, cleaning the bath, in fact any task which requires exertion. Or perhaps you don't do your own cleaning and use a cleaning service. Offering their services for a couple of hours from time to time may make all the difference to your ailing friend.**

- **Making a home-cooked meal, either inviting them to your home or taking the meal to their home. My parents looked after me for two months after I came out of hospital, and it's also enjoyable for carers to have visitors and share a meal with friends to take the pressure off.**

- **Try to do the things you used to do together with your sick friend, e.g., going out to dinner,** the movies, a museum, and taking a stroll in the park. Many activities are still within the reach of heart failure patients, and it's good emotionally for the sick person to feel as much as possible that a conventional life may continue.

- If you do go for a walk with someone whose heart is not pumping as well as yours, be prepared to walk at their rhythm. There is nothing more upsetting and demoralising for someone who cannot keep up the pace. All it does is emphasise the stark contrast between your ability to walk quickly and their inability to do so as they struggle to stay connected to the fit and able person they once were. If you feel like you need a brisk walk, go and exercise on your own before meeting them and then when you do spend time together with those who walk more slowly, you will feel less frustrated at not getting your daily exercise and, more importantly, save their feelings.

- Try asking 'How do you feel today?' rather than 'how are you?' or ignoring the question all together. This gives the impression that you are joining them on the journey to regain their health and do realise that each day may be different. Likewise, there may come a time when they no longer wish for their health to be a matter of conversation, and this is something to be aware of. Although I still have heart failure, I usually say 'I'm holding steady, thank you' when people ask. It's a little expression I learnt from my friend Jeff, and I have found it to be very useful when I have not wished to dwell on my health or go into further detail.

- Avoid such terms as battling or fighting. It implies that they have a choice in the matter and if they don't fight hard enough, then in some way they are responsible for not getting better. I prefer words like 'journey' and 'I'm thinking of you'. The simple act of keeping in touch together with practical help are much more appreciated than battle terminology.

- If you have a cold or the flu, please keep away from your heart patient friends and their family members until you are better. Covid-19 has helped the public to realise the importance of good hand hygiene much more than before, and small changes like social distancing, and sneezing into your elbow or into a tissue which is then discarded may prevent you from spreading germs to someone who is particularly vulnerable.

- Whilst some people are good at expressing how they feel and enjoy giving time and support by their physical presence, some may feel uncomfortable visiting a hospital or a sick person. Maybe it's a fear of their own mortality or perhaps they're squeamish. Sometimes, they just disappear, never to be heard of again. Who knows where they've gone!

- Unfortunately, there may be some people who try to take advantage of your newly vulnerable state. The old adage 'you really know who your friends are when you get sick' often becomes a reality. The sad fact is life goes on around you. You may feel like you are in a state of perpetual slow motion, but the vagaries of modern society remain, and it's important to keep your wits about you.

- Disability remains a powerful and resistant stigma. It's an unfortunate expression and to group everyone into the same category is often unnecessary, limiting, and insensitive. It is essential to take great care in the words used to talk to and describe someone who is now physically challenged.

- As you start to improve it is sometimes preferable not to have to discuss your condition every time you see a visitor. Although, they have not yet found a cure for my illness, I do not want it to define me. At one point, I decided that I would stop calling it an illness and refer to it as a journey. After all, we're all on the same journey through life. It's just that some of us arrive sooner than others and with varying levels of turbulence along the way.

- Some may prefer to show their affection in the giving of gifts. As for me, I've always loved presents. I love to give them, and I love to receive them. For me they represent a symbol of affection and care as well as an indication that someone has been thinking of you. My grandmother was a very generous person and I have always appreciated that quality in others. Gifts don't have to be large or expensive; all gifts are gratefully received and allow the person to feel cherished. Most people think of flowers, grapes, chocolates, or newspapers, but if you wish to be a bit more creative, some of the most thoughtful gifts I have received both within and outside of hospital and which have given me great pleasure may be found on page 242.

Prayers   Hugs   Emails   CDs
Visits   Phone calls   Socks
Text messages   Get well cards
Letters   Teddy bears
Medical research   Balloons   Toothpaste
Shampoo   Flowers   Orchids
Perfume   Bananas
Blueberries   Manicure / Pedicure
Books   DVDs
Magazines
Candles   Dressing gown   Something homemade
Lavender oil
Lap tray   Olive oil   Mini iPad
Blender
Perfumed shower gel   Chocolates   Cookery books

Obviously, it's always prudent to check if the person is allowed to receive flowers as certain hospitals do not permit them. Equally some patients may have dietary restrictions, and some may not be well enough to enjoy some of the items on the list. It took me three years before I could eat chocolate again and a year before I could enjoy receiving a massage.

It's also wonderful to receive gifts even when you are no longer in hospital and heartening to have symbols of love and caring in your home while you're trying to regain your health. I had a fragrant flower garden in one corner of the room that lasted for over a year. Gifts of flowers were constantly replaced, and hardy orchids lasted for months at a time.

The Ring...

While surfing the internet, I came across an interesting concept called 'The Ring'. It was devised by breast cancer survivor and clinical psychologist, Dr. Susan Silk Ph.D., and arbitrator/mediator, Barry Goldman. It's a very simple but helpful premise.

If you draw a circle with several concentric rings, the idea is that those in the middle should receive comfort and are able to unburden to those further out in the rings. The patient is always in the centre of the inner circle and should never be unburdened upon. Likewise, their spouse or carer should be able to receive support from those in the outer rings.

In a similar vein, my friend Virginia believes there are two types of people, 'drains' and 'radiators', and it is very important that the 'drains' do not try to take energy from the patient or their carers while they are in this challenging

3rd Circle of Support

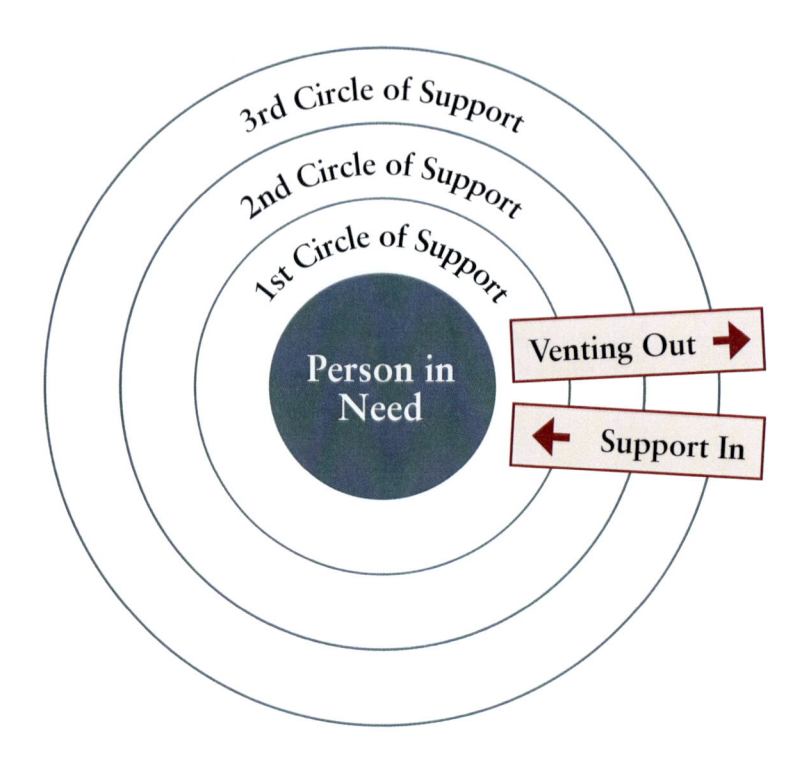

2nd Circle of Support

1st Circle of Support

Person in Need

Venting Out →

← Support In

situation. I have found it quite intriguing that despite knowing that I was seriously ill, people would still try to unburden upon me. I guess, old habits die hard, and if you find yourself in a similar situation my advice would be to keep those energy vampires at a safe distance.

> Many sick people decide not to tell their friends they are ill as it is likely to change fundamentally the whole nature, texture, and subtleties of their relationship. The focus invariably shifts to the illness and smothers the light-heartedness of their former synergy which is often ephemeral and difficult to recapture.

It was very surprising to me that some friends, whom I thought I would always be able to count on, became distant or just disappeared, and others whom I hardly knew, as well as total strangers, were incredibly kind and helpful. I suppose we could put it down to 'fair weather' friendship, but I think it might be more complicated than that. I have spoken with other patients and kindred spirits who have had very similar experiences.

When I lived in Aix-en-Provence as a student at university, a wild wind called *le mistral* would blow for several days and chase the clouds away to reveal a vibrant blue sky and an intense luminosity. Similarly, a near death experience can bring a clarity of thought like the mistral wind chasing the clouds to reveal the light. Sometimes the nuances of life garner enhanced value through suffering, and it is very possible that, when facing a life-threatening illness, not only may friends change, but you may too.

Although it is good to have the support of others, it is also important to be self-reliant. It is all too easy to get bogged down with one's own predicament, become depressed and lose sight of positive changes. After all, if you're always negative you will be no fun to be with and people may no longer wish to spend time with you.

As I have mentioned previously, the first thing I do every day is watch some comedy while I'm eating my breakfast. It's amazing how that release of positive endorphins can help to place you in the right frame of mind for the day ahead.

Other ways to keep your mood elevated include offering to cook someone a meal. It's both creative and an act of love. If you don't know how to cook, try watching cookery shows and/or buy cookery books. Find a recipe you like and keep practising. You will soon find that people will keep coming back if you make delicious food for them.

Take up a hobby, learn a language or a musical instrument. I used to paint when I was at school, but lost touch with that hobby many years ago. I went on a painting course recently and found it very rewarding. Learning to make something or to be creative is extremely important for your well-being. Every time we challenge ourselves and succeed in doing something different our brain secretes a little bit of a magical neurotransmitter called dopamine which gives us a positive feeling and encourages us to want to do it again.

Forgiveness

We can't change everything, but we can change our thoughts. I try not to dwell on the negatives. Sometimes people can be thoughtless but don't always mean to be unkind. Forgiveness is a character trait we can all aspire to. It certainly makes for a more enjoyable life. There are also occasions when people deliberately aim to be unkind but holding on to resentment and anger is never a useful emotion and can become self-destructive, particularly when you already have severe health challenges. Forgiveness is a skill which doesn't always come naturally and may need to be mastered. There is no strict formula, and each situation may require its own unique approach. Furthermore, some situations may never be resolved, but finding peace within yourself and letting go of the hurt may be all that is required to move forward and reclaim a calm and tranquil life.

I remember watching a movie called *The Railway Man* and it compelled me to find out more about the true story behind the film. Eric Lomax, a British officer was captured during the Second World War and was sent to a Japanese POW camp. He was forced to work on the Thai–Burma railway and was tortured by the military secret police for attempting to make a radio. He was eventually rescued by the British Army but even some 30 years later continued to suffer psychological trauma and nightmares from his wartime experiences.

Eric Lomax discovered that one of his torturers, Officer Takashi Nagase, who had worked for the Japanese secret police, was still alive, active in charitable works and had built a Buddhist temple. After hearing about his transformation, Eric Lomax was sceptical, but his wife wrote to Nagase and the reply she received from him was full of compassion.

After the two men corresponded for a while, Lomax travelled with his wife to meet Nagase in Thailand. The humility of Takashi Nagase and Eric Lomax's willingness to forgive enabled both men to move forward with their lives in a positive way. The meeting between these two men is captured in Mike Finlason's documentary *Enemy, My Friend?* and Eric Lomax went on to create 'The Forgiveness Project' which has helped many others.

Eric Lomax's subsequent friendship with Takashi Nagase was a particular inspiration to me in demonstrating the infinite human capacity for forgiveness.

CHAPTER 23

"A little knowledge that acts is worth infinitely more than much knowledge that is idle."

Kahlil Gibran

One thing I have learnt on this journey is that medicine is an inexact science. Whilst modern medicine has made advances in many areas of ill health and there are some cures, treatment for many illnesses, and in particular autoimmunity, remains elusive and is often insufficiently understood. There appears to be very little in a doctor's arsenal to treat these diseases in an acceptable way with few to no side effects.

The current treatment for autoimmune myocarditis is immunosuppressive therapy, e.g., prednisolone, mycophenolate mofetil and cardiac medication. In my own case, I realise that prednisolone was miraculous, and I will remain ever grateful that it saved my life. However, I remember Matthew Manning once telling me that steroids are like loan sharks, they rescue you when you really need them, but your body pays for them dearly in the end! The side effects are often very unpleasant and the longer you remain on the drug, the more severe they can be.

Moreover, one of the most challenging aspects in dealing with such a rare disease has been my interaction with those treating me. I have often admired those who work in the medical profession and have always believed in applying respectful deference to the physician. Throughout my life, I seem to have been surrounded by medicine. From the local village doctor who made house calls and looked after my entire family, to the two physicians I stayed with in France while studying and the multiple medical students I befriended while I lived opposite George Washington Hospital and who lived in my apartment building. These and many similar encounters have left a lasting impression on me. However, whilst I have always thought medicine to be a noble profession, there remains an enormous variation in the quality of care.

Although I admit that, at times, I might have been a challenging patient asking endless questions about my condition etc, whilst some doctors and nurses have been wonderful, others have not understood the complexity of my illness and were loath to admit that they just didn't have all the answers. When you're incredibly sick, you do need empathy, a kind word, a modicum of understanding and agreement to find out more about the case if you simply don't know. In my case, phrases like 'We only usually see this at autopsy' or 'You have a life-threatening illness, we're going to give you lots of nasty drugs now' or 'I'm only interested in what goes on in the UK not the rest of the world' were particularly unhelpful. I have shared with you in writing this book some of the negative interactions that I have experienced, not because I'm dwelling on them but rather to help other medical professionals take a step back from a very sick patient, put themselves in similar shoes and ask themselves what they would like to hear at a time like that. I particularly admire doctors whose egos allow them to reach out to other knowledgeable professionals around the world to ask for their help and advice. We now live in a global world, with internet access which means that good quality communications are immediate. Why struggle when others have perhaps already trodden a similar path?

I would humbly suggest that you should not feel concerned or guilty if you have reached the end of the road with one doctor. If you find that you are no longer making progress, or the doctor's emphasis has shifted to other matters, sometimes a change to someone else who might have different ideas, is still interested and curious about finding a cure or better treatment might be all you need.

> **As I have mentioned in Chapter 18, the heart is a wonderful but highly complex organ. Whilst most cardiologists are interventionists, unblocking arteries, putting in new valves, etc, the effect of the emotions and subconscious on the heart is little understood. In my opinion and as a distillation of my own experience, what you say to a patient can have just as much effect as any drug.**

Self-Help

So, what can you do if you have received the life-changing diagnosis of myocarditis with associated heart failure and cardiomyopathy? Medication is often essential, but it can only do so much. I have therefore attempted to find ways which might help improve symptoms and empower you to take a more active role in your health and well-being. As mentioned before, please seek medical advice when starting something new as each person may have differing needs and not all methods may be appropriate.

When I was first ill, very few cardiologists were able to guide me in the complementary therapies and nutrition which exist to help heart patients. I have therefore summarised below some of the therapies that I have tried to help me on this journey.

Education

As I have already mentioned at the beginning of Part Two, it is essential that you learn all you can about the heart and the intricacies of your own individual cardiac problems. This information will empower you and allow you to play an important role in conversations with medical staff. Furthermore, the knowledge you obtain may help to reduce anxiety and give you a better perspective in the decision-making process.

Nutrition

It is hard to believe that so little is learnt in medical school about nutrition. Many doctors receive a very superficial level of training in this important aspect of the human body and are therefore rarely able to give you up-to-date advice on diet and nutrition to help your condition, despite knowing that partaking in unhealthy living may exacerbate or worsen cardiovascular disease.

I have mentioned throughout the book the importance of maintaining sufficient levels of vitamin D, magnesium, omega-3 and eating a low-salt, anti-inflammatory diet. Whilst I am not an expert, there are now many excellent books on this subject, written in detail by numerous nutritionists and functional doctors. It would therefore seem essential to learn all you can about how certain nutrient-dense foods may help to improve your overall well-being as well as your cardiac health (for further details see Chapters 20 and 21).

Recent studies suggest that intermittent fasting (e.g., where you fast for 16 hours a day and eat only during the remaining 8 hours) may be a useful tool in controlling weight, lowering blood pressure, reducing cholesterol, and controlling diabetes. However, one word of caution, particularly if your heart is already damaged: fasting may lead to an electrolyte imbalance which may render the heart unstable and prone to arrhythmias.

Another area of concern is crash dieting. It is now believed that a sudden deterioration in heart function may occur following a very low-calorie diet. The sudden drop in calories may cause fat to be released into the blood stream and taken up by the heart muscle. This sudden excess of fat worsens the heart's function and may lead to serious problems. Therefore, it is essential to check with your doctor before starting intermittent fasting and/or a very low-calorie diet.

Exercise

Studies suggest that gentle exercise is good for the heart (except, of course, when you are suffering from acute myocarditis). However, there is increasing evidence that marathons, extreme endurance sports and excessive exercise may be deleterious to the heart. If there are any underlying heart conditions, genetic or otherwise, they will usually present themselves when the heart is put under intense pressure in this way.

Generally in the body, blood flow is laminar. However, under conditions of high flow, particularly in the ascending aorta, laminar flow can be disrupted and become turbulent. High intensity exercise causes blood to flow in non-laminar columns through vessels which may damage their delicate walls and cause microscopic tears. Consequently this means that instead of the blood flowing along in one direction you get columns that thrash about left and right and in all directions, a bit like water in the ocean during a storm.

Studies have looked at runners and found that their troponin T levels have often been elevated at the end of marathons. Troponin T is a marker in the blood for heart muscle damage. As we have a set number of heart muscle cells (myocytes) in a lifetime, damaging them on a regular basis would not seem prudent. Basketball, extreme cycling, and marathon running have been shown to be particularly problematic, and a number of young, fit athletes have died following such extreme endeavours. Many studies have shown that under extreme pressure the right ventricle expands, and the left ventricle becomes smaller. This remodelling of the heart is usually temporary in young people and will revert after about a week to ten days, but as the athlete increases in age, the heart does not bounce back as easily, and it appears to age the heart prematurely.

In my own experience I have found walking, swimming, yoga and pilates to be excellent ways to keep my body moving whilst taking care of my heart. Furthermore, scientific studies show increasingly that spending time amidst trees may produce manifold physical and psychological benefits.

Supplements

I find it helpful to have my minerals and vitamins checked regularly to make sure that I am not deficient in any important elements. When the heart is damaged, there may be an increased requirement for certain supplements to ensure the heart is working optimally.

I discovered a fascinating book called *The Metabolic Heart* written by Dr. Stephen Sinatra, an eminent cardiologist, and it contains many cardiac-specific suggestions to maintain a healthy heart including, D-ribose, CoQ10, L-carnitine, together with my favourite supplement, magnesium.

Each person will have different needs and working with a nutritionist and/or a functional doctor may help point you in the right direction.

Earthing/Grounding

You may remember in Chapter 16 that I was advised by Father Ignacio to walk on the ground barefoot while I was in Argentina. I had never heard of this concept before and was intrigued to find out why that might make a difference to my heart. Whilst it is not yet in the mainstream, grounding or earthing has been the subject of much research as to its positive effects on inflammation, the immune response, wound healing, the prevention of autoimmune and chronic inflammatory diseases, pain, and sleep.

We often forget that we are electrical beings. The earth has a constant negative charge, and our bodies build up a positive charge because we are not frequently in direct and uninterrupted contact with the earth. The simple act of grounding oneself daily can even out this positive charge and return the body to a more neutral state. It also appears to have a positive impact on the viscosity of the blood which is an important factor in cardiovascular disease.

Unfortunately, in the modern world, we often spend vast periods of time out of contact with the earth's surface and in the last 50 years we have often worn synthetic or rubber-soled shoes which insulate us from the benefits of earthing. Weeks and months may go by without grounding. This is also now often the case for children who hardly ever run about on the grass barefoot, spending the day from waking until bedtime totally insulated from the earth's surface. Most adults and children only very rarely walk barefoot on a regular basis except perhaps on the beach while they are on holiday. I have often contemplated why I always felt and looked so refreshed after spending much of my holiday in the sea and walking along the sand. It's certainly an interesting concept, and I have been surprised by how many people in the older generation from many different countries already appear to be aware of the benefits of earthing. It certainly has no side effects, is free and anything that can reduce inflammation can only be beneficial.

For more information you may wish to explore the work of Clinton Ober and Dr. Stephen Sinatra (an eminent cardiologist) who together wrote a book called *Earthing: The Most Important Health Discovery Ever?*

Hypnosis

I first discovered hypnosis many years ago when I had a bout of insomnia. After reading a sign in my local pharmacy for a practitioner, I decided to give it a whirl. It worked like a charm, and I have used it from time to time to help me reach a deep level of relaxation.

Many people have strong opinions about hypnosis and don't believe they could ever be hypnotised. However, it is my understanding that the hypnotherapist merely acts as a conduit for you to connect with your own subconscious on a much deeper level. You are always in control.

It is thought that hypnosis activates the right brain and promotes a deep state of relaxation while the left brain dials down its activity. Gentle language with focus on breath and body may be all that is needed for you to achieve this trance-like state, and invariably just a half-hour session may give the feeling of a full night's slumber.

Osteopathy

Amusingly, the founder of osteopathy, Dr. Andrew Taylor Still, was quoted as having said 'The only type of person who would not benefit from osteopathy is a dead one!'

The benefits of osteopathy have long been documented. Osteopaths are highly trained experts in the musculoskeletal system (muscles, joints and associated tissues) and its relationship to other systems of the body. Osteopaths believe that a problem with one system or part of the anatomy affects the entirety of the human body and its ability to heal itself. Osteopathy may have positive effects on the immune system and help with insomnia. It may also alleviate pain, promote relaxation and is known to reduce stress levels by increasing the efficiency of the body's systems such as blood flow, nerve supply and the immune system.

Psychotherapy

In my opinion, psychotherapy may be very helpful in cases of chronic illness, but it is essential to find the most complementary match. I remember starting out on this journey with someone who just sat opposite me and repeated throughout the hour-long session 'And how does that make you feel?' I didn't find that approach very helpful and was hoping to find someone more analytical and able to give practical suggestions. Then out of the blue, a new therapist was recommended to me. She had been through and recovered from a long-term illness and was able to draw on her own experience to make practical suggestions and offer helpful explanations. It turned out to be a much better fit for my personality. Therefore, my conclusion would be if you're not happy with the first therapist, keep looking.

Maintenance

The importance of learning how to look after yourself is essential when you have been diagnosed with heart failure. This means learning how to avoid the constant merry go round of a hospital admission, getting stabilised in the hospital environment, being released, only to be re-admitted within 6 weeks with the same symptoms of severe shortness of breath, swollen ankles, and oedema. After about two years of struggling to manage my heart failure, I received a booklet produced by Intermountain Healthcare entitled *Living with Heart Failure*. This booklet has proved to be invaluable to me. Up until that point, no one had ever told me that I should weigh myself daily, that I should reduce my salt to 2 grams daily and minimise my fluid intake to 64 fluid ounces per day. I have included some extracts from the booklet in Chapter 19 but I would strongly recommend that anyone suffering from heart failure obtain a copy directly from Intermountain Healthcare as it is full of essential information about managing your heart health.

My Tips to Maintain a Healthy Heart

1. Avoid Chronic Stress
2. Daily Comedy
3. Daily Magnesium
4. Drink Minimal Alcohol
5. Eat a Low Salt Diet
6. Listen to Music
7. Nourishment, - spiritual and wholesome food
8. Peace and Quiet, whether by taking time to be alone, as well as yoga, meditation, and hypnosis
9. Set aside time during the day to be Internet-free
10. Sleep without IT equipment next to your bed
11. Stop Smoking
12. Sunlight
13. Surround yourself with Positive People
14. Take Gentle exercise, outside preferably somewhere green, but no marathons or extreme exercise
15. Walk barefoot on the ground or on sand

CHAPTER 24

"Natural forces within us are the true healers of disease."

Hippocrates

It's very easy, in this modern world, to get caught up in a toxic working environment and not realise the toll it is taking on one's health. As mentioned before, I have always had a strong work ethic and had pursued an interesting international career. However, my genteel upbringing and 'intuitive-sensitive' personality type had not prepared me for much of the Machiavellian behaviour that we so often encounter in the corporate world and the constant stress of these environments.

With the benefit of hindsight, the physical warning signs were there. Whilst I tried to seek remedies for my various ailments, the origin of most of my issues was stress-related.

Many people have asked me the cause of my illness. There is no doubt that there was probably a final trigger, the domino which toppled all the others. There is a term which I have discovered from my research into stress. It is known as the 'allostatic load' which is the 'wear and tear on the body' which accumulates as an individual is exposed to repeated or chronic stress. The term was introduced by Bruce McEwen and Eliot Stellar in 1993 and represents the physiological consequences of chronic exposure to fluctuating or heightened neural or neuroendocrine response which results from repeated or prolonged chronic stress. You have no doubt heard about the fight or flight response which in cases of chronic stress is constantly activated and leads to adrenal exhaustion.

I believe this played a strong part in what happened to me and this, along with many factors, provided the perfect terrain to allow an opportunistic virus to trigger the development of myocarditis. A number of these factors may include:

- Chronic low vitamin D levels
- Chronic low ferritin levels
- Chronic stress and adrenal exhaustion
- Deficiency of magnesium
- Deficiency of omega-3
- Deficiency of zinc
- Hormonal imbalance
- High inflammation in the body
- High-salt diet
- Leaky gut syndrome
- Raynaud's syndrome
- Undiagnosed gluten intolerance

All these elements affect the functioning of the immune system and may also have a deleterious impact on the heart.

It doesn't help that the speed of modern life seems to be increasing at such a pace that the brain is having difficulty keeping up. This has been greatly amplified by the advent of technologies such as the internet and social media. It is fascinating to see how different age groups are coping with this phenomenon. There are those who have passed through an age which started with the simple manual typewriter, then progressed to the electric typewriter using paper with carbon paper copies or stencils to make multiple copies. We then moved onto mainframe computers, personal computers and more recently laptops, tablets, and smartphones. There are others who have only lived in the internet age and are often less able to cope without their multiple hand-held devices, sometimes succumbing to the dangers of clickbait and algorithms which lead to programmed addiction.

Whilst the internet age is more convenient in many ways, this has also meant that managers are encroaching increasingly on employees' 'free time'. They often feel more and more pressured to check emails and text messages on a frequent basis, before, during and after the working day, during weekends and vacations just to keep up and stay ahead of the curve. Any resistance to this expectation is often viewed as not being committed to the job.

Sometimes the body rebels against this hypervigilant state and succumbs to this chronic stress through illness and, in severe cases, death. The Japanese even have a term for it, *karoshi*, which can be translated literally as 'overwork death'. The human body is not a machine, and the deeper question should be asked as to why we are here – is it just to work and make money for someone else, or should we strive to enjoy life, free of guilt and take pleasure in kindness to others?

It is indeed unfortunate that we now endure a much more stressful existence in all aspects of life. Not only do we encounter much more stress in the workplace with the expectation of completing vast amounts of work in an increasingly short time following the change in work practices with the internet, but we are also expected to do the work of many people as we carry out our daily lives.

I have listed below some examples:
- Letters and invoices are no longer sent by mail but via email and need to printed using your own time, printer, ink, and paper.
- Travelling involves similar preparation of boarding passes, loading luggage onto a conveyor belt and printing off one's own luggage tags.
- Self-service in restaurants and cafes where you sometimes become the chef and waiter/waitress.
- Self-service in supermarkets and petrol stations where you become the check-out assistant and garage attendant.
- Online banking, often fine for simple transactions but almost impossible for anything more complicated.
- Endless phone calls to call centres for a variety of tasks which often take hours to complete.

It is hardly surprising considering the stressful situation in which I found myself that my body took its own intervention – *'You're not listening so I'm going to make you listen'* and I was catapulted out of that stressful environment, never to return.

There is no doubt that some people are now beginning to realise the harm that social media, the internet and 24-hour news are doing to our society. Some believe that it is so harmful and distractive that they have deleted social media from their computers and phones. It seems a pity that some are missing out on life around them, staring at their phones and not communicating with others. They're not fully in the moment. Some studies even show that just the mere presence of a phone on a table between two people, without it even being used – negatively affects the interaction.

Likewise, if you are spending time with someone and all they do is look at their phone, their behaviour gives the impression that they're bored of your company and would rather be communicating with someone else. Ironically if they met that same person, they would probably repeat this same behaviour by ignoring the person in front of them and communicate with you on their smartphone.

It's now almost impossible to walk in the street without someone bumping into you whilst staring intently at their smartphones. It seems that even a simple walk cannot be carried out without the security of a handheld device. Often some people appear to be more comfortable communicating by text and social media than talking face-to-face or on the phone.

I see people around me struggling to keep up. Some friends have even been to the doctor to check whether they have problems with their memories. The sheer quantity of information which we are trying to juggle in our short-term memory is making us feel like we have early onset Alzheimer's. Interestingly, since I stopped this intense activity, my memory has improved enormously and I no longer have a constant twitching muscle under my eye, rather like Herbert Lom as Chief Inspector Dreyfus in the *Pink Panther* movies – not a good look.

> Whilst the advent of smartphones, tablets and computers has provided us with immeasurable benefits, I believe that moderation is key in ensuring that the impact on our bodies is a positive one. It is also essential to have periods in life when we take time out to retreat for reflection. If we don't treasure those moments to truly stop and experience life, then it is easy to pass through life and never really experience it at all.

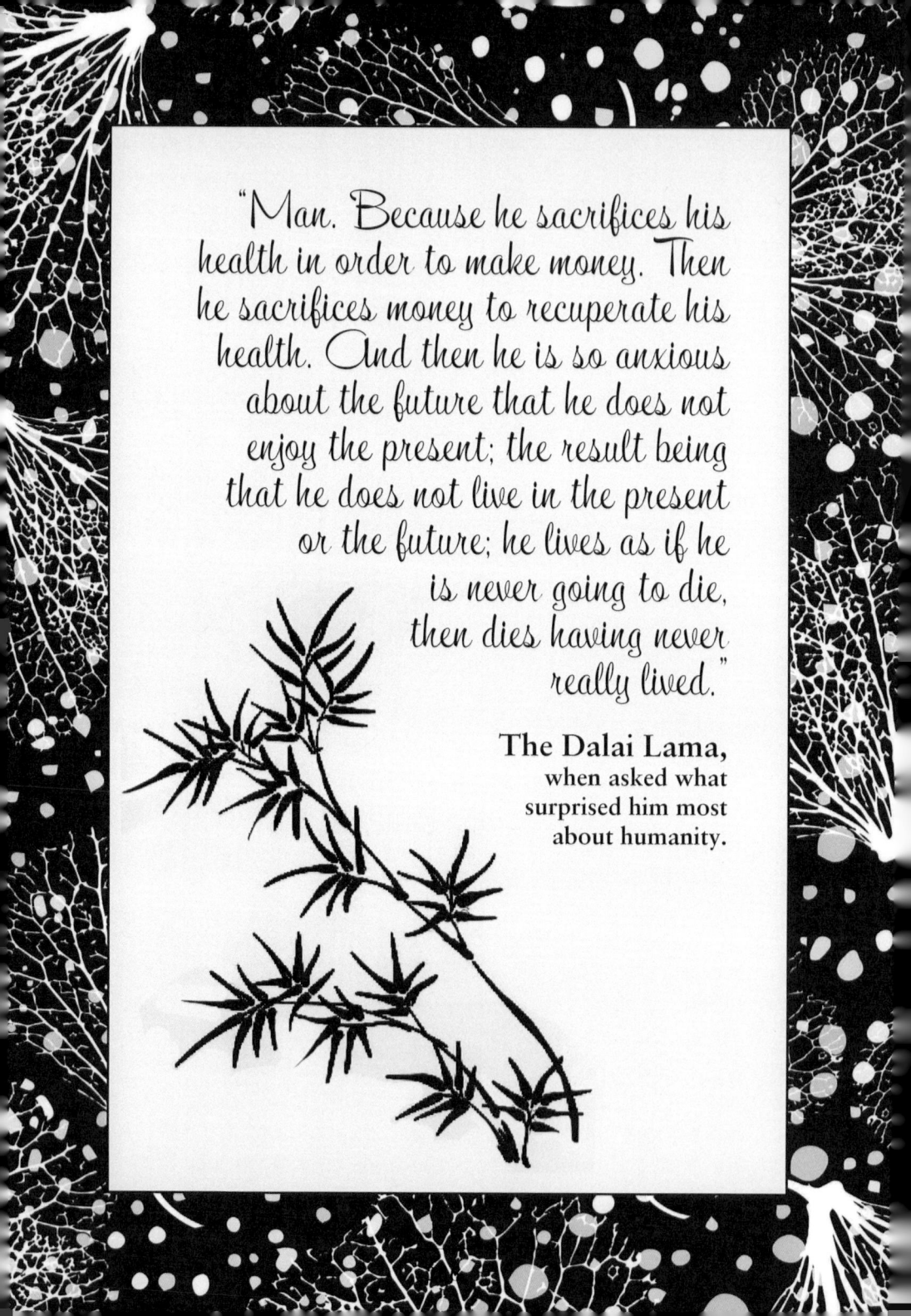

"Man. Because he sacrifices his health in order to make money. Then he sacrifices money to recuperate his health. And then he is so anxious about the future that he does not enjoy the present; the result being that he does not live in the present or the future; he lives as if he is never going to die, then dies having never really lived."

The Dalai Lama, when asked what surprised him most about humanity.

CHAPTER 25

"I think cinema, movies, and magic have always been closely associated. The very earliest people who made film were magicians."

Francis Ford Coppola

As you might have noticed, I just love movies. Watching a good movie provokes all kinds of emotions. Even if you watch a movie with others, it often remains a solitary, personal experience, and may make a memorable visual and auditory impact on you which lasts a whole lifetime. The way we feel about love has often been shaped by movies, and sometimes just hearing a solitary phrase within a dialogue that touches you deeply may make watching the entire movie worthwhile.

Movies often have a magical way of speaking to you, catching you unawares, touching you in ways you never thought possible. Emotions you thought were individual to you may be analysed and brought into the open, and your own hurt may be overcome as you realise others have shared a similar path. The combination of powerful words, visuals and accompanying music may open you up and may even set you on a different path. For some, watching a movie is a form of pure escapism, entertainment, and stress relief, but for others it may act as a form of therapy, sometimes known as 'cinetherapy', helping the viewer to come to terms with many of life's challenges.

I grew up in a small village and at that time a gift from my grandmother of a small black and white TV in my bedroom was my only personal portal to the rest of the world. I used to spend hours in bed late at night watching hilarious Woody Allen movies when I should have been sleeping. Now we have 24-hour access to a plethora of varied entertainment. However, for me, movies have not lost any of their magic.

One of my favourite film directors was Nora Ephron. She had a magical ability to capture some of the most wonderful, heartfelt moments on film. One of her favourite phrases was 'everything is copy', and she inspired me to collect some of the phrases which people have uttered to me over the years, kind and unkind, and I have worked some of these into this manuscript.

If you are looking for a good movie, I have listed below some of my favourites which have touched and stayed with me. Some are funny, some moving and some exciting. However, you won't find any horror movies included in the list as I prefer to protect my little heart. Enjoy!

A Family Man
A Fish Called Wanda
A Rainy Day in New York
A Star is Born (original)
Amélie
American Beauty

Burn After Reading
Catch Me if You Can
Chariots of Fire
Chocolat
Cinema Paradiso
Crazy Rich Asians

Crouching Tiger, Hidden Dragon
Claire's Knee
Dallas Buyers Club
Dave
Dead Again
Deep Waters
Dream Horse
Downton Abbey
Erin Brokovitch
Everything is Copy
Eye in the Sky
Flight
Forrest Gump
Four Weddings and a Funeral
Fracture
Gigi
Green Book
Good Will Hunting
Haute Cuisine
Hello, My Name is Doris
Il Postino
It's a Wonderful Life
It's Complicated
Jean de Florette
Julie & Julia
Juliet's Letters
Les Emotifs Anonymes
Les Visiteurs
Life is Beautiful
Little Miss Sunshine
Lion
Manhattan Murder Mystery
Manon des Sources
Matchpoint
Muriel's Wedding
My Big Fat Greek Wedding
My Life as a Dog
Notting Hill
No Way Out
Orlando
Out of Africa
PS I Love You
Perfumes

Rabbit-Proof Fence
Rear Window
Searching for Sugarman
Something's Gotta Give
Sleeper
Sleepless in Seattle
Sliding Doors
Slumdog Millionaire
Steel Magnolias
St. Elmo's Fire
The Artist
The Bank Job
The Big Short
The Bodyguard
The Bourne Ultimatum
The Curious Case of Benjamin Button
The Dish
The Elephant Man
The Graduate
The Great Gatsby (original)
The Green Mile
The Holiday
The Hundred-Foot Journey
The King's Speech
The Kite Runner
The Lincoln Lawyer
The Lover
The Lunch Box
The Morning Show
The Queen's Gambit
The Railway Man
The Silent Child
The Sixth Sense
The Story of the Weeping Camel
There's Something About Mary
Three Billboards Outside Ebbing Missouri
Toy Story
Under the Tuscan Sun
Waking Ned
What We Did on our Holidays
When Harry Met Sally
You've Got Mail

CHAPTER 26

"Someone is sitting in the shade today because someone planted a tree a long time ago."

Warren Buffett

In the relatively few years since the onset of my illness, the world of medicine has moved forward considerably. Medical practitioners are now embracing the internet, and it is much easier to find a plethora of information from reliable sources than it was when I was lying in my hospital bed several years ago. There are numerous websites and podcasts which I consult on a regular basis, and I have listed some of them overleaf in alphabetical order for your interest and information.

References are provided for informational purposes only and do not constitute endorsement of any websites, products, or other sources. I also cannot vouch for the absoluteness of my suggestions. Please seek professional medical advice before buying or utilising any product. Readers should be aware that the websites listed in this book may change.

Helpful Websites

actiononsalt.org.uk
americanheart.org
bhf.org.uk
bloodpressureuk.org
bsh.org.uk
campbellteaching.co.uk - Dr. John Campbell
cardiogauge.com – Dr. Nathan Ritter
cardiomyopathy.org
childrenscardiomyopathy.org
cim.umaryland.edu
clinicaltrials.gov
dietdoctor.com - Dr. David Unwin
discoveringosteopathy.vhx.tv
escardio.org
health.clevelandclinic.org
heart.bmj.com
heartmdinstitute.com – Dr. Stephen T. Sinatra
hfsa.org
ifm.org – Dr. Mark Harman
intermountinghealthcare.org
mayoclinic.org
medscape.com
myocarditisfoundation.org – Dr. Leslie T. Cooper
myocarditisuk.com
nutritionalmagnesiumassociation.org
stewartnutrition.co.uk – Dr. Alan Stewart
yorkcardiology.co.uk – Dr. Sanjay Gupta

Bibliography

In the process of writing *The Unexpected* I have been inspired by and, in some cases, have referred to the work of other writers. Where I have quoted directly, the attributions are in the main body of the text but there are also writings listed here that I would like to mention that gave me inspiration or that I enjoyed:

Coping with Prednisolone, Eugenia Zukerman and Julie R. Ingelfinger, MD, St. Martin's Press, 2007

Deadly Medicine, Thomas J. Moore, Simon & Schuster, 1995

Dragon Slippers, Rosalind B. Penfold, Harper Press, 2006

Food: What the Heck Should I Cook? Mark Harman, MD, Little Brown Spark, 2019

Highly Intuitive People, Heidi Sawyer, Hay House, 2015

I Feel Bad About My Neck and Other Thoughts on Being a Woman, Nora Ephron, Doubleday, 2006

Join-Up: Horse Sense for People, Monty Roberts, Harper Collins, 2001

Les Très Riches Heures de Mrs Mole, Ronald Searle, Harper Collins Publishers, 2011

Myocarditis: From Bench to Bedside, Leslie T. Cooper, Jr. MD, Humana Press, 2013

Reclaim Health, Dr. David Beales, Janice Benning, Helen Whitten, Julia MacDonald, Dr. Gina Johnson, July 2019

Simply Raymond, Raymond Blanc, Headline Publishing Group, 2021

The Diabetes Weight-Loss Cookbook, Katie and Giancarlo Caldesi, Kyle Books, 2019

The Grateful Heart: Diary of a Heart Transplant, Candace C. Moose, Rosalie Ink Publications, 2005

The Health Equation: A Way of Life, Gerry Gajadharsingh, BookBaby 2014

The Heart of Leonardo, Francis C. Wells, Springer, 2013

The Idiot Brain, Dean Burnett, Guardian Books, 2016

The Life-Changing Magic of Tidying, Marie Kondo, Vermilion, 2014

The Magnesium Miracle, Dr. Carolyn Dean, MD, ND, Vintage, 2017

The Power of Nice, Linda Kaplan Thaler and Robin Koval, Virgin Books, 2016

The Sinatra Solution, Stephen T. Sinatra, MD, FACC, FACN, CNS, Basic Health Publications, 2011

Your Mind Can Heal Your Body, Matthew Manning, Piatkus, 2011

Used with Kind Permission

Logo: by kind permission of the Myocarditis Foundation

Image: 'The Notting Hill Bookshop'
by kind permission of the company.

'Living with Heart Failure', Intermountain Healthcare
extracted by kind permission of the organisation.

'Salt's Effects on your Body', Blood Pressure UK
extracted by kind permission of the organisation.

Picture Credits

End Papers	Scene of Bariloche Llao Llao from Argentinian money/Adobe Stock Photo
Cover, iv,	Weimaraner/Adobe Stock Photo
ix–x, 156–157, 180	Chiyogami Paper/Adobe Stock Photo
85	LifeVest/Zoll Medical Corporation
107	Heart Clip Art/Cliparto
160	Leonardo da Vinci/Science Photo Library
194–198	Living with Heart Failure/Intermountain Healthcare
Ribbon Heart	Red Heart/Adobe Stock Photo (Special Edition only)

All other photographs are courtesy of the author.

About the Author

Kayte Alexander studied French language, literature, and civilisation at the University of Aix-en-Provence in the South of France. After working at several international organisations in Brussels and Washington, DC, she moved to London to work in the City, the financial district of London. This is her first book.

BARILOCHE LLAO-LLAO